Medical Pharmacology at a Glance

Medical Pharmacology at a Glance

Michael J. Neal

Emeritus Professor of Pharmacology
King's College London
London

Sixth edition

WILEY-BLACKWELL

A John Wiley & Sons, Ltd., Publication

This edition first published 2009 © 1987, 1992, 1997, 2002, 2005, 2009 by Michael J. Neal

Blackwell Publishing was acquired by John Wiley & Sons in February 2007. Blackwell's publishing program has been merged with Wiley's global Scientific, Technical and Medical business to form Wiley-Blackwell.

Registered office: John Wiley & Sons Ltd, The Atrium, Southern Gate, Chichester, West Sussex, PO19 8SQ, UK

Editorial offices: 9600 Garsington Road, Oxford, OX4 2DQ, UK
The Atrium, Southern Gate, Chichester, West Sussex, PO19 8SQ, UK
111 River Street, Hoboken, NJ 07030-5774, USA

For details of our global editorial offices, for customer services and for information about how to apply for permission to reuse the copyright material in this book please see our website at www.wiley.com/wiley-blackwell

Library of Congress Cataloging-in-Publication Data
Neal, M. J.
    Medical pharmacology at a glance / Michael J. Neal. — 6th ed.
        p. ; cm.
    Includes bibliographical references and index.
    ISBN 978-1-4051-8197-6
    1. Clinical pharmacology.   I. Title.
    [DNLM: 1. Pharmacology, Clinical. QV 38 N342m 2009]
    RM301.28.N43 2009
    615′.1—dc22
                                                    2008039513

ISBN: 978-1-4051-8197-6

A catalogue record for this book is available from the British Library.

Set in 9/11.5pt Times by Graphicraft Limited, Hong Kong
Printed and bound in Singapore by Ho Printing Singapore Pte Ltd

2   2011

Contents

Preface

This book is written primarily for medical students but it should also be useful to students and scientists in other disciplines who would like an elementary and concise introduction to pharmacology.

In this book the text has been reduced to a minimum for understanding the figures. Nevertheless, I have attempted in each chapter to explain how the drugs produce their effects and to outline their uses.

In this sixth edition the chapters have been updated. The chapter on antifungal and antiviral drugs has been divided into two separate chapters to allow these topics to be dealt with in a little more detail. However, the most obvious change is that this latest edition is in full colour. I hope this will not only make the figures more attractive but will make them clearer and easier to understand. Another innovation in this latest edition is the addition of 'case studies'.

Acknowledgements

I am grateful to Professor M. Marbur, Professor J.M. Ritter and Professor P.J. Ciclitira for their advice and helpful comments on the case studies relevant to their special interests.

How to use this book

Each of the chapters (listed on page 5) represents a particular topic, corresponding roughly to a 60-minute lecture. Beginners in pharmacology should start at Chapter 1 and first read through the text on the left-hand pages (which occasionally continues to the facing right-hand page above the ruled line) of several chapters, using the figures only as a guide.

Once the general outline has been grasped, it is probably better to concentrate on the *figures* one at a time. Some are quite complicated and certainly cannot be taken in 'at a glance'. Each should be studied carefully and worked through together with the legends (right-hand pages). Because many drugs appear in more than one chapter, considerable cross-referencing has been provided. As progress is made through the book, use of this cross-referencing will provide valuable reinforcement and a greater understanding of drug action. Once the information has been understood, the figures should subsequently require little more than a brief look to refresh the memory.

The figures are highly diagrammatic and not to scale.

Further reading

British National Formulary. British Medical Association and The Royal Pharmaceutical Society of Great Britain, London (about 900 pp). The BNF is updated twice a year.

Rang, H.P., Dale, M.M., Ritter, J.M. & Flower, R.J. (2007) *Pharmacology*, 5th edn, Churchill Livingstone, Edinburgh (829 pp).

Bennett, P.N. & Brown, M.J. (2008) *Clinical Pharmacology*, 10th edn, Churchill Livingstone, Edinburgh (694 pp).

1 Introduction: principles of drug action

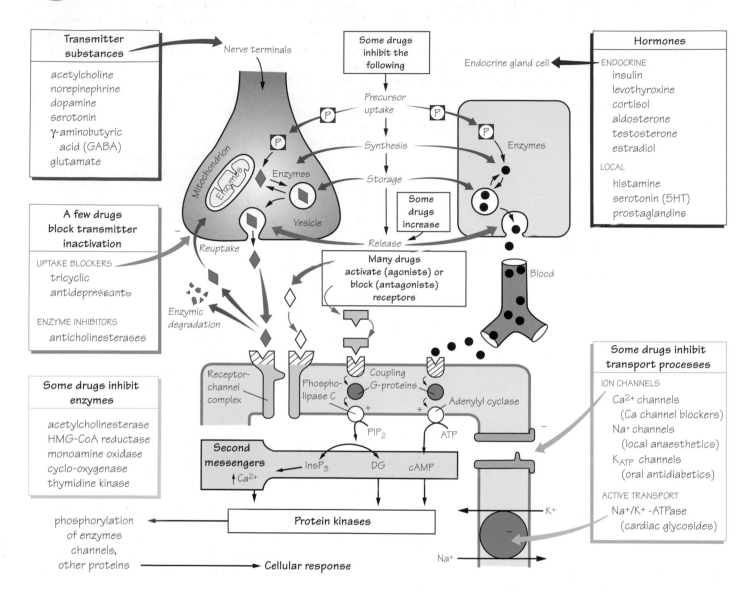

Medical pharmacology is the science of chemicals (drugs) that interact with the human body. These interactions are divided into two classes:

- **pharmacodynamics** – the effects of the drug on the body; and
- **pharmacokinetics** – the way the body affects the drug with time (i.e. absorption, distribution, metabolism and excretion).

The most common ways in which a drug can produce its effects are shown in the figure. A few drugs (e.g. activated charcoal, osmotic diuretics) act by virtue of their physicochemical properties, and this is called **non-specific** drug action. Some drugs act as false substrates or inhibitors for certain **transport systems** (bottom right) or **enzymes** (bottom left). However, most drugs produce their effects by acting on specific protein molecules, usually located in the cell membrane. These proteins are called **receptors** (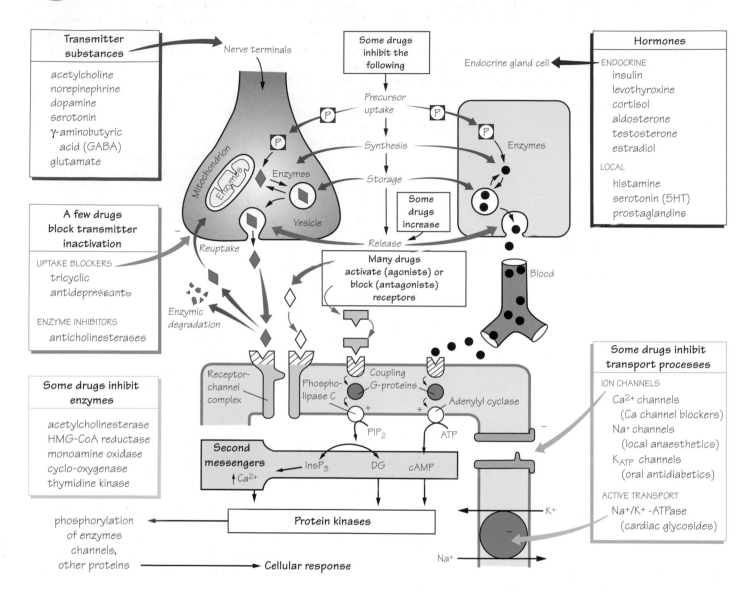), and they normally respond to endogenous chemicals in the body. These chemicals are either synaptic **transmitter substances** (top left, ♦) or **hormones** (top right, ●). For example, acetylcholine is a transmitter substance released from motor nerve endings; it activates receptors in skeletal muscle, initiating a sequence of events that results in contraction of the muscle. Chemicals (e.g. acetylcholine) or drugs that activate receptors and produce a response are called **agonists** (◇). Some drugs, called **antagonists** (▽), combine with receptors, but do not activate them. Antagonists reduce the probability of the transmitter substance (or another agonist) combining with the receptor and so reduce or block its action.

The activation of receptors by an agonist or hormone is coupled to the physiological or biochemical responses by transduction mechanisms (lower figure) that often (but not always) involve molecules called 'second messengers' (▭).

The interaction between a drug and the binding site of the receptor depends on the complementarity of 'fit' of the two molecules. The closer the fit and the greater the number of bonds (usually noncovalent), the stronger will be the attractive forces between them, and the higher the **affinity** of the drug for the receptor. The ability of a drug to combine with one particular type of receptor is called **specificity**. No drug is truly specific, but many have a relatively **selective** action on one type of receptor.

Drugs are prescribed to produce a therapeutic effect, but they often produce additional **unwanted effects** (Chapter 46) that range from the trivial (e.g. slight nausea) to the fatal (e.g. aplastic anaemia).

Receptors

These are protein molecules that are normally activated by transmitters or hormones. Many receptors have now been cloned and their amino acid sequences determined. The four main types of receptor are listed below.

1 Agonist (ligand)-gated ion channels are made up of protein subunits that form a central pore (e.g. nicotinic receptor, Chapter 6; γ-aminobutyric acid (GABA) receptor, Chapter 24).

2 G-protein-coupled receptors (see below) form a family of receptors with seven membrane-spanning helices. They are linked (usually) to physiological responses by second messengers.

3 Nuclear receptors for steroid hormones (Chapter 34) and thyroid hormones (Chapter 35) are present in the cell nucleus and regulate transcription and thus protein synthesis.

4 Kinase-linked receptors are surface receptors that possess (usually) intrinsic tyrosine kinase activity. They include receptors for insulin, cytokines and growth factors (Chapter 36).

Transmitter substances are chemicals released from nerve terminals that diffuse across the synaptic cleft and bind to the receptors. This binding activates the receptors by changing their conformation, and triggers a sequence of postsynaptic events resulting in, for example, muscle contraction or glandular secretion. Following its release, the transmitter is inactivated (left of figure) by either enzymic degradation (e.g. acetylcholine) or reuptake (e.g. norepinephrine [noradrenaline], GABA). Many drugs act by either reducing or enhancing synaptic transmission.

Hormones are chemicals released into the bloodstream; they produce their physiological effects on tissues possessing the necessary specific hormone receptors. Drugs may interact with the endocrine system by inhibiting (e.g. antithyroid drugs, Chapter 35) or increasing (e.g. oral antidiabetic agents, Chapter 36) hormone release. Other drugs interact with hormone receptors, which may be activated (e.g. steroidal anti-inflammatory drugs, Chapter 33) or blocked (e.g. oestrogen antagonists, Chapter 34). Local hormones (autacoids), such as histamine, serotonin (5-hydroxytryptamine, 5HT), kinins and prostaglandins, are released in pathological processes. The effects of histamine can sometimes be blocked with antihistamines (Chapter 11), and drugs that block prostaglandin synthesis (e.g. aspirin) are widely used as anti-inflammatory agents (Chapter 32).

Transport systems

The lipid cell membrane provides a barrier against the transport of hydrophilic molecules into or out of the cell.

Ion channels are selective pores in the membrane that allow the ready transfer of ions down their electrochemical gradient. The open–closed state of these channels is controlled either by the membrane potential (voltage-gated channels) or by transmitter substances (ligand-gated channels). Some channels (e.g. Ca^{2+} channels in the heart) are both voltage and transmitter gated. Voltage-gated channels for sodium, potassium and calcium have the same basic structure (Chapter 5), and subtypes exist for each different channel. Important examples of drugs that act on voltage-gated channels are *calcium-channel blockers* (Chapter 16), which block L-type calcium channels in vascular smooth muscle and the heart, and *local anaesthetics* (Chapter 5), which block sodium channels in nerves. Some *anticonvulsants* (Chapter 25) and some *antiarrhythmic* drugs (Chapter 17) also block Na^+ channels. No clinically useful drug acts primarily on voltage-gated K^+ channels, but *oral antidiabetic* drugs act on a different type of K^+ channel that is regulated by intracellular adenosine triphosphate (ATP, Chapter 36).

Active transport processes are used to transfer substances against their concentration gradients. They utilize special carrier molecules in the membrane and require metabolic energy. Two examples are listed below.

1 *Sodium pump*. This expels Na^+ ions from inside the cell by a mechanism that derives energy from ATP and involves the enzyme adenosine triphosphatase (ATPase). The carrier is linked to the transfer of K^+ ions into the cell. The *cardiac glycosides* (Chapter 18) act by inhibiting the Na^+/K^+-ATPase. Na^+ and/or Cl^- transport processes in the kidney are inhibited by some *diuretics* (Chapter 14).

2 *Norepinephrine transport*. The *tricyclic antidepressants* (Chapter 28) prolong the action of norepinephrine by blocking its reuptake into central nerve terminals.

Enzymes

These are catalytic proteins that increase the *rate* of chemical reactions in the body. Drugs that act by inhibiting enzymes include: *anticholinesterases*, which enhance the action of acetylcholine (Chapters 6 and 8); *carbonic anhydrase inhibitors*, which are diuretics (i.e. increase urine flow, Chapter 14); *monoamine oxidase inhibitors*, which are antidepressants (Chapter 28); and inhibitors of *cyclo-oxygenase* (e.g. aspirin, Chapter 32).

Second messengers

These are chemicals whose intracellular concentration increases or, more rarely, decreases in response to receptor activation by agonists, and which trigger processes that eventually result in a cellular response. The most studied second messengers are: Ca^{2+} ions, cyclic adenosine monophosphate (cAMP), inositol-1,4,5-trisphosphate ($InsP_3$) and diacylglycerol (DG).

cAMP is formed from ATP by the enzyme adenylyl cyclase when, for example, β-adrenoceptors are stimulated. The cAMP activates an enzyme (protein kinase A), which phosphorylates a protein (enzyme or ion channel) and leads to a physiological effect.

$InsP_3$ and DG are formed from membrane phosphatidylinositol 4,5-bisphosphate by activation of a phospholipase C. Both messengers can, like cAMP, activate kinases, but $InsP_3$ does this indirectly by mobilizing intracellular calcium stores. Some muscarinic effects of acetylcholine and $α_1$-adrenergic effects involve this mechanism (Chapter 7).

G-proteins

G-protein-coupled receptors are linked to their responses by a family of regulatory guanosine triphosphate (GTP)-binding proteins (G-proteins). The receptor–agonist complex induces a conformational change in the G-protein, causing its α-subunit to bind GTP. The α–GTP complex dissociates from the G-protein and activates (or inhibits) the membrane enzyme or channel. The signal to the enzyme or channel ends because α–GTP has intrinsic GTPase activity and turns itself off by hydrolysing the GTP to guanosine diphosphate (GDP). α–GDP then reassociates with the βγ G-protein subunits.

2 Drug–receptor interactions

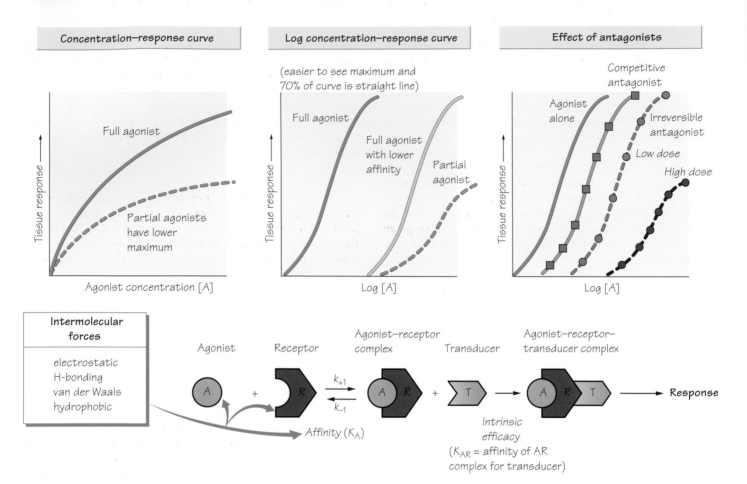

The tissues in the body have only a few basic responses when exposed to agonists (e.g. muscle contraction, glandular secretion), and the quantitative relationship between these physiological responses and the concentration of the agonist can be measured by using **bioassays**. The first part of the drug–receptor interaction, i.e. the **binding of drug to receptor**, can be studied in isolation using **binding assays**.

It has been found by experiment that, for many tissues and agonists, when the response is plotted against the concentration of the drug, a curve is produced that is often hyperbolic (**concentration–response curve**, top left). In practice, it is often more convenient to plot the response against the logarithm of the agonist concentration (**log concentration–response curve**, middle top). Assuming that the interaction between the drug (A) and the receptor (R) (lower figure) obeys the law of mass action, then the concentration of the drug–receptor complex (AR) is given by:

$$[AR] = \frac{[R_O][A]}{K_D + [A]}$$

where R_O = total concentration of receptors, A = agonist concentration, K_D = dissociation constant and AR = concentration of occupied receptors.

As this is the equation for a hyperbola, the shape of the dose–response curve is explained if the response is directly proportional to $[AR]$. Unfortunately, this simple theory does not explain another experimental finding – some agonists, called **partial agonists**, cannot elicit the same maximum response as full agonists even if they have the same affinity for the receptor (top left and middle, ━ ━). Thus, in addition to having affinity for the receptor, an agonist has another chemical property, called **intrinsic efficacy**, which is its ability to elicit a response when it binds to a receptor (lower figure).

A **competitive antagonist** has no intrinsic efficacy and, by occupying a proportion of the receptors, effectively dilutes the receptor concentration. This causes a parallel shift of the log concentration–response curve to the right (top right, ■), but the maximum response is not depressed. In contrast, **irreversible antagonists** depress the maximum response (top right, ●). However, at low concentrations, a parallel shift of the log concentration–response curve may occur without a reduction in the maximum response (top right, ●). Because an irreversible antagonist in effect removes receptors from the system, it is clear that not all of the receptors need to be occupied to elicit the maximum response (i.e. there is a **receptor reserve**).

Binding of drugs to receptors

Intermolecular forces

Drug molecules in the environment of receptors are attracted initially by relatively long-range electrostatic forces. Then, if the molecule is suitably shaped to fit closely to the binding site of the receptor, hydrogen bonds and van der Waals forces briefly bind the drug to the receptor. Irreversible antagonists bind to receptors with strong covalent bonds.

Affinity

This is a measure of how avidly a drug binds to its receptor. It is characterized by the equilibrium dissociation constant (K_D), which is the ratio of rate constants for the reverse (k_{-1}) and forward (k_{+1}) reactions between the drug and the receptor. The reciprocal of K_D is called the affinity constant (K_A), and (in the absence of receptor reserve, see below) is the concentration of drug that produces 50% of the maximum response.

Antagonists

Most antagonists are drugs that *bind to receptors but do not activate them*. They may be competitive or irreversible. Other types of antagonist are less common.

Competitive antagonists bind reversibly with receptors, and the tissue response can be returned to normal by increasing the dose of agonist, because this increases the probability of agonist–receptor collisions at the expense of antagonist–receptor collisions. The ability of higher doses of agonist to overcome the effects of the antagonist results in a parallel shift of the dose–response curve to the right and is the hallmark of competitive antagonism.

Irreversible antagonists have an effect that cannot be reversed by increasing the concentration of agonist. The only important example is *phenoxybenzamine*, which binds covalently with α-adrenoceptors. The resulting insurmountable block is valuable in the management of phaeochromocytoma, a tumour that releases large amounts of epinephrine (adrenaline).

Other types of antagonism

Non-competitive antagonists do not bind to the receptor site but act downstream to prevent the response to an agonist, e.g. calcium-channel blockers (Chapter 15).

Chemical antagonists simply bind to the active drug and inactivate it; e.g. protamine abolishes the anticoagulant effect of heparin (Chapter 19).

Physiological antagonists are two agents with opposite effects that tend to cancel one another out, e.g. prostacyclin and thromboxane A_2 on platelet aggregation (Chapter 19).

Receptor reserve

In some tissues (e.g. smooth muscle), irreversible antagonists initially shift the log dose–response curve to the right without reducing the maximum response, indicating that the maximum response can be obtained without the agonist occupying all the receptors. The excess receptors are sometimes called 'spare' receptors, but this is a misleading term because they are of functional significance. They increase both the sensitivity and speed of a system because the concentration of drug–receptor complex (and hence the response) depends on the product of the agonist concentration and the *total* receptor concentration.

Partial agonists

These are agonists that cannot elicit the same maximum response as a 'full' agonist. The reasons for this are unknown. One suggestion is that agonism depends on the affinity of the drug–receptor complex for a *transducer molecule* (lower figure). Thus, a full agonist produces a complex with high affinity for the transducer (e.g. the coupling G-proteins, Chapter 1), whereas a partial agonist–receptor complex has a lower affinity for the transducer and so cannot elicit the full response.

When acting alone at receptors, partial agonists stimulate a physiological response, but they can antagonize the effects of a full agonist.

This is because some of the receptors previously occupied by the full agonist become occupied by the partial agonist, which has a smaller effect (e.g. some β-adrenoceptor antagonists, Chapters 15 and 16).

Intrinsic efficacy

This is the ability of an agonist to alter the conformation of a receptor in such a way that it elicits a response in the system. It is defined as the affinity of the agonist–receptor complex for a transducer.

Partial agonists and receptor reserve. A drug that is a partial agonist in a tissue with no receptor reserve may be a full agonist in a tissue possessing many 'spare' receptors, because its poor efficacy can be offset by activating a larger number of receptors than that required by a full agonist.

Bioassay

Bioassays involve the use of a biological tissue to relate drug concentration to a physiological response. Usually isolated tissues are used because it is then easier to control the drug concentration around the tissue and reflex responses are abolished. However, bioassays sometimes involve whole animals, and the same principles are used in clinical trials.

Bioassays can be used to estimate:
- the concentration of a drug (largely superseded by chemical methods);
- its binding constants; or
- its potency relative to another drug.

Measurement of the relative potencies of a series of agonists on different tissues has been one of the main ways used to classify receptors, e.g. adrenoceptors (Chapter 7).

Binding assays

Binding assays are simple and very adaptable. Membrane fragments from homogenized tissues are incubated with radiolabelled drug (usually ^3H) and then recovered by filtration. After correction for non-specific binding, the [^3H]drug bound to the receptors can be determined and estimations made of K_A and B_{max} (number of binding sites). Binding assays are widely used to study drug receptors, but have the disadvantage that no functional response is measured, and often the radiolabelled drug does not bind to a single class of receptor.

Localization of receptors

The distribution of receptors, e.g. in sections of the brain, can be studied using autoradiography. In humans, positron-emitting drugs can sometimes be used to obtain images (positron emission tomography [PET] scanning) showing the location and density of receptors, e.g. dopamine receptors in the brain (Chapter 27).

Tachyphylaxis, desensitization, tolerance and drug resistance

When a drug is given repeatedly, its effects often decrease with time. If the decrease in effect occurs quickly (minutes), it is called **tachyphylaxis** or desensitization. **Tolerance** refers to a slower decrease in response (days or weeks). **Drug resistance** is a term reserved for the loss of effect of chemotherapeutic agents, e.g. antimalarials (Chapter 43). Tolerance may involve increased metabolism of a drug, e.g. ethanol, barbiturates (Chapter 3), or homeostatic mechanisms (usually not understood) that gradually reduce the effect of a drug, e.g. morphine (Chapter 29). Changes in receptors may cause desensitization, e.g. suxamethonium (Chapter 6). A decrease in receptor number (downregulation) can lead to tolerance, e.g. insulin (Chapter 36).

3 Drug absorption, distribution and excretion

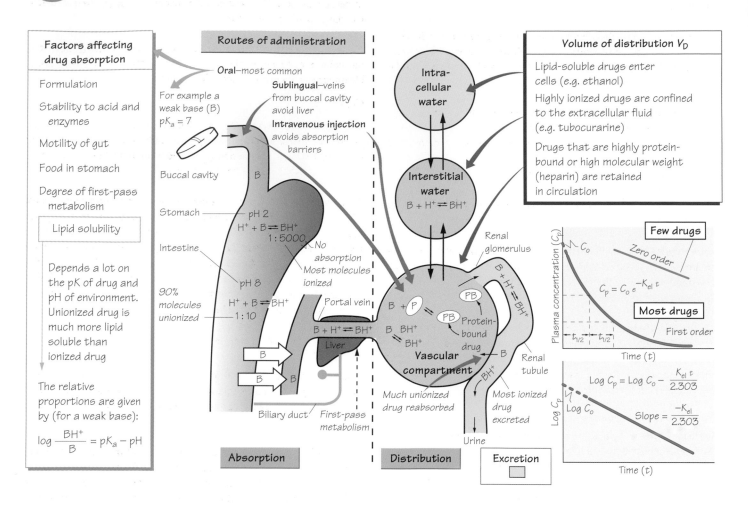

Most drugs are given **orally** and they must pass through the gut wall to enter the bloodstream (left of figure, ⇨). This **absorption** process is affected by many factors (left), but is usually proportional to the **lipid solubility** of the drug. Thus, the absorption of non-ionized molecules (B) is favoured because the latter are far more lipid soluble than ionized molecules (BH+), which are surrounded by a 'shell' of water molecules. Drugs are absorbed mainly from the small intestine because of the latter's large surface area. This is true even for weak acids (e.g. aspirin), which are non-ionized in the acid (HCl) of the stomach. Drugs absorbed from the gastrointestinal tract enter the portal circulation (left, ▨) and some are extensively metabolized as they pass through the liver (first-pass metabolism).

Drugs that are sufficiently lipid soluble to be readily absorbed orally are rapidly distributed throughout the body water compartments (◯). Many drugs are loosely bound to plasma albumin, and an equilibrium forms between the bound (PB) and free (B) drug in the plasma. Drug that is bound to plasma proteins is confined to the vascular system and cannot exert its pharmacological actions.

If a drug is given by **intravenous injection**, it enters the blood and is rapidly distributed to the tissues. By taking repeated blood samples, the fall in plasma concentration of the drug with time (i.e. the rate of drug elimination) can be measured (right, top graph). Often the concentration falls rapidly at first, but then the rate of decline progressively decreases. Such a curve is called **exponential**, and this means that, at any given time, a **constant fraction** of the drug present is eliminated in unit time. Many drugs show an exponential fall in plasma concentration because the rates at which the drug elimination processes work are themselves usually proportional to the concentration of drug in the plasma. The following processes are involved.

1 Elimination in the urine by glomerular filtration (right, ▨).
2 Metabolism, usually by the liver.
3 Uptake by the liver and subsequent elimination in the bile (——— solid line from liver).

A process that depends on the concentration at any given time is called **first** order; most drugs exhibit first-order elimination kinetics. If any enzyme system responsible for drug metabolism becomes **saturated**, then the elimination kinetics change to **zero order**, i.e. the rate of elimination proceeds at a constant rate and is unaffected by an increased concentration of the drug (e.g. ethanol, phenytoin).

Routes of administration

Drugs can be administered orally or parenterally (i.e. by a nongastrointestinal route).

Oral Most drugs are absorbed by this route and, because of its convenience, it is the most widely used. However, some drugs (e.g. benzylpenicillin, insulin) are destroyed by the acid or enzymes in the gut and must be given parenterally.

Intravenous injection The drug directly enters into the circulation and bypasses the absorption barriers. It is used:
- where a rapid effect is required (e.g. furosemide in pulmonary oedema);
- for continuous administration (infusion);
- for large volumes; and
- for drugs that cause local tissue damage if given by other routes (e.g. cytotoxic drugs).

Intramuscular and subcutaneous injections Drugs in aqueous solution are usually absorbed fairly rapidly, but absorption can be slowed by giving the drug in the form of an ester (e.g. antipsychotic depot preparations, Chapter 27).

Other routes These include **inhalation** (e.g. volatile anaesthetics, some drugs used in asthma) and **topical** (e.g. ointments). **Sublingual** and **rectal** administration avoids the portal circulation, and sublingual preparations in particular are valuable in administering drugs subject to a high degree of first-pass metabolism.

Distribution and excretion

Distribution around the body occurs when the drug reaches the circulation. It must then penetrate tissues to act.

The $t_{1/2}$ (**half-life**) is the time taken for the concentration of drug in the blood to fall by half its original value (right, top graph). Measurement of $t_{1/2}$ allows the calculation of the *elimination rate constant* (K_{el}) from the formula:

$$K_{el} = \frac{0.69}{t}$$

where K_{el} is the fraction of drug present at any time that would be eliminated in unit time (e.g. $K_{el} = 0.02$ min^{-1} means that 2% of the drug present is eliminated in 1 min).

The exponential curve of plasma concentration (C_p) against time (t) is described by:

$$C_p = C_0 e^{-K_{el}t}$$

where C_0 = the initial apparent plasma concentration. By taking logarithms, the exponential curve can be transformed into a more convenient straight line (right, bottom graph) from which C_0 and $t_{1/2}$ can readily be determined.

Volume of distribution (V_D) This is the apparent volume into which the drug is distributed. Following an intravenous injection:

$$V_D = \frac{\text{dose}}{C_0}$$

A value of $V_D < 5$ L implies that the drug is retained within the vascular compartment. A value of < 15 L suggests that the drug is restricted to the extracellular fluid, whereas large volumes of distribution ($V_D > 15$ L) indicate distribution throughout the total body water or concentration in certain tissues. The volume of distribution can be used to calculate the *clearance* of the drug.

Clearance This is an important concept in pharmacokinetics. It is the volume of blood or plasma cleared of drug in unit time. Plasma clearance (Cl_p) is given by the relationship:

$$Cl_p = V_D K_{el}$$

The rate of elimination = $Cl_p \times C_p$. Clearance is the sum of individual clearance values. Thus, $Cl_p = Cl_m$ (metabolic clearance) + Cl_r (renal excretion). Clearance, but not $t_{1/2}$, provides an indication of the ability of the liver and kidney to dispose of drugs.

Drug dosage Clearance values can be used to plan dosage regimens. Ideally, in drug treatment, a steady-state plasma concentration (C_{pss}) is required within a known therapeutic range. A steady state will be achieved when the rate of drug entering the systemic circulation (dosage rate) equals the rate of elimination. Thus, the dosing rate = $Cl \times C_{pss}$. This equation could be applied to an intravenous infusion because the entire dose enters the circulation at a known rate. For oral administration, the equation becomes:

$$\frac{F \times \text{dose}}{\text{dosing interval}} = Cl_p \times C_p, \text{ average}$$

where F = *bioavailability* of the drug. The $t_{1/2}$ value of a drug is useful in choosing a dosing interval that does not produce excessively high peaks (toxic levels) and low troughs (ineffective levels) in drug concentration.

Bioavailability This is a term used to describe the proportion of administered drug reaching the systemic circulation. Bioavailability is 100% following an intravenous injection ($F = 1$), but drugs are usually given orally, and the proportion of the dose reaching the systemic circulation varies with different drugs and also from patient to patient. Drugs subject to a high degree of first-pass metabolism may be almost inactive orally (e.g. glyceryl trinitrate, lidocaine).

Excretion

Renal excretion This is ultimately responsible for the elimination of most drugs. Drugs appear in the glomerular filtrate, but if they are lipid soluble they are readily reabsorbed in the renal tubules by passive diffusion. Metabolism of a drug often results in a less lipid-soluble compound, aiding renal excretion (see Chapter 4).

The ionization of weak acids and bases depends on the pH of the tubular fluid. Manipulation of the urine pH is sometimes useful in increasing renal excretion. For example, bicarbonate administration makes the urine alkaline; this ionizes aspirin, making it less lipid soluble and increasing its rate of excretion.

Weak acids and weak bases are actively secreted in the proximal tubule. Penicillins, eg thiazide diuretics, morphine.

Biliary excretion Some drugs (e.g. diethylstilbestrol) are concentrated in the bile and excreted into the intestine where they may be reabsorbed. This enterohepatic circulation increases the persistence of a drug in the body.

4 Drug metabolism

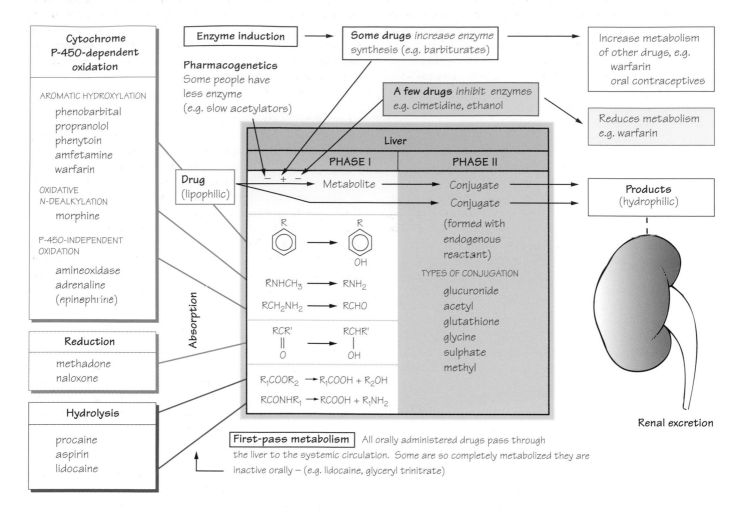

Drug metabolism has two important effects.

1 The drug is made more **hydrophilic** – this hastens its excretion by the kidneys (right, ▨) because the less lipid-soluble metabolite is not readily reabsorbed in the renal tubules.

2 The metabolites are usually **less active** than the parent drug. However, this is not always so, and sometimes the metabolites are as active as (or more active than) the original drug. For example, diazepam (a drug used to treat anxiety) is metabolized to nordiazepam and oxazepam, both of which are active. **Prodrugs** are inactive until they are metabolized in the body to the active drug. For example, levodopa, an antiparkinsonian drug (Chapter 26), is metabolized to dopamine, whereas the hypotensive drug methyldopa (Chapter 15) is metabolized to α-methylnorepinephrine.

The **liver** is the main organ of drug metabolism and is involved in two general types of reaction.

Phase I reactions These involve the biotransformation of a drug to a more polar metabolite (left of figure) by introducing or unmasking a functional group (e.g. –OH, –NH₂, –SH).

Oxidations are the most common reactions and these are catalysed by an important class of enzymes called the mixed function oxidases (**cytochrome P-450s**). The substrate specificity of this enzyme complex is very low and many different drugs can be oxidized (examples, top left). Other phase I reactions are **reductions** (middle left) and **hydrolysis** (bottom left).

Phase II reactions Drugs or phase I metabolites that are not sufficiently polar to be excreted rapidly by the kidneys are made more hydrophilic by conjugation with endogenous compounds in the liver (centre of figure).

Repeated administration of some drugs (top) increases the synthesis of cytochrome P-450 (**enzyme induction**). This increases the rate of metabolism of the inducing drug and also of other drugs metabolized by the same enzyme (top right). In contrast, drugs sometimes **inhibit** microsomal enzyme activity (top, ▨) and this increases the action of drugs metabolized by the same enzyme (top right, ☐).

In addition to these drug–drug interactions, the metabolism of drugs may be influenced by **genetic factors** (pharmacogenetics), age and some diseases, especially those affecting the liver.

Drugs

A few drugs (e.g. gallamine, Chapter 6) are highly polar because they are fully ionized at physiological pH values. Such drugs are metabolized little, if at all, and the termination of their actions depends mainly on renal excretion. However, most drugs are highly lipophilic and are often bound to plasma proteins. As the protein-bound drug is not filtered at the renal glomerulus and the free drug readily diffuses back from the tubule into the blood, such drugs would have a very prolonged action if their removal relied on renal excretion alone. In general, drugs are metabolized to more polar compounds, which are more easily excreted by the kidneys.

Liver

The main organ of drug metabolism is the liver, but other organs, such as the gastrointestinal tract and lungs, have considerable activity. Drugs given orally are usually absorbed in the small intestine and enter the portal system to travel to the liver, where they may be extensively metabolized (e.g. lidocaine, morphine, propranolol). This is called *first-pass metabolism*, a term that does not refer only to hepatic metabolism. For example, chlorpromazine is metabolized more in the intestine than by the liver.

Phase I reactions

The most common reaction is *oxidation*. Other, relatively uncommon, reactions are *reduction* and *hydrolysis*.

Microsomal mixed function oxidase system

Many of the enzymes involved in drug metabolism are located on the smooth endoplasmic reticulum, which forms small vesicles when the tissue is homogenized. These vesicles can be isolated by differential centrifugation and are called microsomes.

Microsomal drug oxidations involve nicotinamide–adenine dinucleotide phosphate (reduced form) (NADPH), oxygen and two key enzymes: (i) a flavoprotein, NADPH-cytochrome P-450 reductase; and (ii) a haemoprotein, cytochrome P-450, which acts as a terminal oxidase. Numerous (CYP) isoforms of P-450 exist with different, but often overlapping, substrate specificities. About half a dozen P-450 isoforms account for most hepatic drug metabolism. CYP3A4 is worth remembering because it metabolizes more than 50% of drugs.

Phase II reactions

These usually occur in the liver and involve conjugation of a drug or its phase I metabolite with an endogenous substance. The resulting conjugates are almost always less active and are polar molecules that are readily excreted by the kidneys.

Factors affecting drug metabolism

Enzyme induction

Some drugs (e.g. *phenobarbital*, *carbamazepine*, *ethanol* and, especially, *rifampicin*) and pollutants (e.g. *polycyclic aromatic hydrocarbons* in tobacco smoke) increase the activity of drug-metabolizing enzymes. The mechanisms involved are unclear, but the chemicals somehow cause specific DNA sequences to 'switch on' the production of the appropriate enzyme(s), usually one or more cytochrome P-450 subtypes. However, not all enzymes subject to induction are microsomal. For example, hepatic alcohol dehydrogenase occurs in the cytoplasm.

Enzyme inhibition

Enzyme inhibition may cause adverse drug interactions. These interactions tend to occur more rapidly than those involving enzyme induction because they occur as soon as the inhibiting drug reaches a high enough concentration to compete with the affected drug. Drugs may inhibit different forms of cytochrome P-450 and so affect the metabolism only of drugs metabolized by that particular isoenzyme. *Cimetidine* inhibits the metabolism of several potentially toxic drugs including phenytoin, warfarin and theophylline. *Erythromycin* also inhibits the cytochrome P-450 system and increases the activity of theophylline, warfarin, carbamazepine and digoxin.

Genetic polymorphisms

The study of how genetic determinants affect drug action is called *pharmacogenetics*. The response to drugs varies between individuals and, because the variations usually have a Gaussian distribution, it is assumed that the determinant of the response is multifactorial. However, some drug responses show discontinuous variation and, in these cases, the population can be divided into two or more groups, suggesting a single-gene polymorphism. For example, about 8% of the population have faulty expression of CYP2D6, the P-450 isoform responsible for debrisoquine hydroxylation. These poor hydroxylators show exaggerated and prolonged responses to drugs such as propranolol and metoprolol (Chapter 15), which undergo extensive hepatic metabolism.

Drug-acetylating enzymes

Hepatic *N*-acetylase displays genetic polymorphism. About 50% of the population acetylate isoniazid (an antitubercular drug) rapidly, whereas the other 50% acetylate it slowly. Slow acetylation is caused by an autosomal recessive gene that is associated with decreased hepatic *N*-acetylase activity. Slow acetylators are more likely to accumulate the drug and to experience adverse reactions.

Plasma pseudocholinesterase

Rarely, (< 1:2500) a deficiency of this enzyme occurs and this extends the duration of action of suxamethonium (a frequently used neuromuscular blocking drug) from about 6 min to over 2 h or more.

Age

Hepatic microsomal enzymes and renal mechanisms are reduced at birth, especially in preterm babies. Both systems develop rapidly during the first 4 weeks of life. There are various methods for calculating paediatric doses (see *British National Formulary*).

In the elderly, hepatic metabolism of drugs may be reduced, but declining renal function is usually more important. By 65 years, the glomerular filtration rate (GFR) decreases by 30%, and every following year it falls a further 1–2% (as a result of cell loss and decreased renal blood flow). Thus, older people need smaller doses of many drugs than do younger persons, especially centrally acting drugs (e.g. opioids, benzodiazepines, antidepressants), to which the elderly seem to become more sensitive (by unknown changes in the brain).

Metabolism and drug toxicity

Occasionally, reactive products of drug metabolism are toxic to various organs, especially the liver. *Paracetamol*, a widely used weak analgesic, normally undergoes glucuronidation and sulphation. However, these processes become saturated at high doses and the drug is then conjugated with glutathione. If the glutathione supply becomes depleted, then a reactive and potentially lethal hepatotoxic metabolite accumulates (Chapter 45).

5 Local anaesthetics

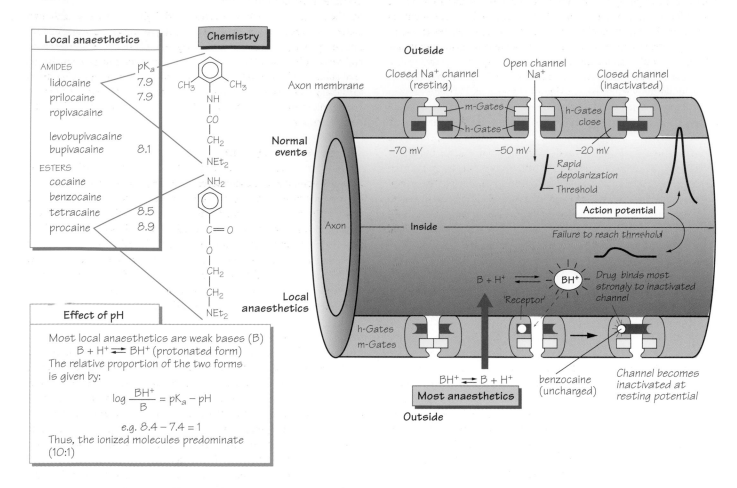

Local anaesthetics (top left) are drugs used to prevent pain by causing a reversible block of conduction along nerve fibres. Most are weak bases that exist mainly in a protonated form at body pH (bottom left). The drugs penetrate the nerve in a non-ionized (lipophilic) form (➡) but, once inside the axon, some ionized molecules (☼) are formed and these block the **Na⁺ channels** (☐) preventing the generation of **action potentials** (lower half of figure).

All nerve fibres are sensitive to local anaesthetics but, in general, small-diameter fibres are more sensitive than large fibres. Thus, a **differential block** can be achieved where the smaller pain and autonomic fibres are blocked, whereas coarse touch and movement fibres are spared. Local anaesthetics vary widely in their potency, duration of action, toxicity and ability to penetrate mucous membranes.

Local anaesthetics depress other excitable tissues (e.g. myocardium) if the concentration in the blood is sufficiently high, but their main unwanted systemic effects involve the central nervous system. **Lidocaine** is the most widely used agent. It acts more rapidly and is more stable than most other local anaesthetics. When given with epinephrine, its action lasts about 90 min. **Prilocaine** is similar to lidocaine, but is more extensively metabolized and is less toxic in equipotent doses. **Bupivacaine** has a slow onset (up to 30 min) but a very long duration of action, up to 8 h when used for nerve blocks. It is often used in pregnancy to produce continuous epidural blockade during labour. It is also the main drug used for spinal anaesthesia in the UK. **Benzocaine** is a neutral, water-insoluble local anaesthetic of low potency. Its only use is in **surface anaesthesia** for non-inflamed tissue (e.g. mouth and pharynx). The more toxic agents, **tetracaine** and **cocaine**, have restricted use. Cocaine is primarily used for surface anaesthesia where its intrinsic vasoconstrictor action is desirable (e.g. in the nose). Tetracaine drops are used in ophthalmology to anaesthetize the cornea, but less toxic drugs such as **oxybupro-caine** and **proxymetacaine**, which cause much less initial stinging, are better.

Hypersensitivity reactions may occur with local anaesthetics, especially in atopic patients, and more often with procaine and other esters of *p*-aminobenzoic acid.

Na⁺ channels

Excitable tissues possess special voltage-gated Na⁺ channels that consist of one large glycoprotein α-subunit and sometimes two smaller β-subunits of unknown function. The α-subunit has four identical domains, each containing six membrane-spanning α-helices (S1–S6). The 24 cylindrical helices are stacked together radially in the membrane to form a central channel. Exactly how voltage-gated channels work is not known, but their conductance (gNa^+) is given by $gNa^+ = \bar{g}Na^+m^3h$, where $\bar{g}Na^+$ is the maximum conductance possible, and m and h are gating constants that depend on the membrane potential. In the figure, these constants are shown schematically as physical gates within the channel. At the resting potential, most h-gates (blue) are open and the m-gates (yellow) are closed (closed channel). Depolarization causes the m-gates to open (open channel), but the intense depolarization of the action potential then causes the h-gates to close the channel (inactivation). This sequence is shown in the upper half of the figure (left to right). The m-gate may correspond to the four positively charged S4 helices, which are thought to open the channel by moving outwards and rotating in response to membrane depolarization. The h-gate responsible for inactivation may be the intracellular loop connecting the S3 and S5 helices; this swings into the internal mouth of the channel and closes it.

Action potential

If enough Na⁺ channels are opened, then the rate of Na⁺ entry into the axon exceeds the rate of K⁺ exit, and at this point, the threshold potential, entry of Na⁺ ions further depolarizes the membrane. This opens more Na⁺ channels, resulting in further depolarization, which opens more Na⁺ channels, and so on. The fast inward Na⁺ current quickly depolarizes the membrane towards the Na⁺ equilibrium potential (around + 67 mV). Then, inactivation of the Na⁺ channels and the continuing efflux of K⁺ ions cause repolarization of the membrane. Finally, the Na⁺ channels regain their normal 'excitable' state and the Na⁺ pump restores the lost K⁺ and removes the gained Na⁺ ions.

Mechanism of local anaesthetics

Local anaesthetics *penetrate* into the interior of the axon in the form of the lipid-soluble free base. There, protonated molecules are formed, which then enter and *plug* the Na⁺ channels after binding to a '*receptor*' (residues of the S6 transmembrane helix). Thus, quaternary (fully protonated) local anaesthetics work only if they are injected inside the nerve axon. Uncharged agents (e.g. benzocaine) dissolve in the membrane, but the channels are blocked in an all-or-none manner. Thus, ionized and non-ionized molecules act in essentially the same way (i.e. by binding to a 'receptor' on the Na⁺ channel). This 'blocks' the channel, largely by preventing the opening of h-gates (i.e. by increasing inactivation). Eventually, so many channels are inactivated that their number falls below the minimum necessary for depolarization to reach threshold and, because action potentials cannot be generated, nerve block occurs. Local anaesthetics are 'use dependent' (i.e. the degree of block is proportional to the rate of nerve stimulation). This indicates that more drug molecules (in their protonated form) enter the Na⁺ channels when they are open and cause more inactivation.

Chemistry

Commonly used local anaesthetics consist of a lipophilic end (often an aromatic ring) and a hydrophilic end (usually a secondary or tertiary amine), connected by an intermediate chain that incorporates an ester or amide linkage.

Unwanted effects

Central nervous system

Synthetic agents produce sedation and light-headedness, although anxiety and restlessness sometimes occur, presumably because central inhibitory synapses are depressed. Higher toxic doses cause twitching and visual disturbances, whereas severe toxicity causes convulsions and coma, with respiratory and cardiac depression resulting from medullary depression. Even cocaine, which has central stimulant properties unrelated to its local anaesthetic action, may cause death by respiratory depression.

Cardiovascular system

With the exception of cocaine, which causes vasoconstriction – by blocking norepinephrine (noradrenaline) reuptake – local anaesthetics cause vasodilatation, partly by a direct action on the blood vessels and partly by blocking their sympathetic nerve supply. The result of vasodilatation and myocardial depression is a decrease in blood pressure, which may be severe, especially with bupivacaine. The $R(-)$-stereoisomer of bupivacaine, levobupivacaine may be less cardiotoxic than racemic bupivacaine because the $R(-)$-isomer has less affinity for myocardial Na⁺ channels than does the $S(+)$-isomer. Ropivacaine is a single (S)-isomer and may also have reduced cardiotoxicity.

Duration of action

In general, high potency and long duration are related to high lipid solubility because this results in much of the locally applied drug entering the cells. Vasoconstriction also tends to prolong the anaesthetic effect by reducing systemic distribution of the agent, and this can be achieved by the addition of a vasoconstrictor, such as epinephrine (adrenaline) or, less often, norepinephrine. Vasoconstrictors must not be used to produce ring-block of an extremity (e.g. finger or toe) because they may cause prolonged ischaemia and gangrene.

Amides are dealkylated in the liver, and esters (not cocaine) are hydrolysed by plasma pseudocholinesterase; however, drug metabolism has little effect on the duration of action of agents actually in the tissues.

Methods of administration

Surface anaesthesia

Topical application to external or mucosal surfaces.

Infiltration anaesthesia

Subcutaneous injection to act on local nerve endings, usually with a vasoconstrictor.

Nerve block

Techniques range from infiltration of anaesthetic around a single nerve (e.g. dental anaesthesia) to epidural and spinal anaesthesia. In spinal anaesthesia (intrathecal block), a drug is injected into the cerebrospinal fluid in the subarachnoid space. In epidural anaesthesia, the anaesthetic is injected outside the dura. Spinal anaesthesia is technically far easier to produce than epidural anaesthesia, but the latter technique virtually eliminates the postanaesthetic complications, such as headache.

Intravenous regional anaesthesia

Anaesthetic is injected intravenously into an exsanguinated limb. A tourniquet prevents the agent from reaching the systemic circulation.

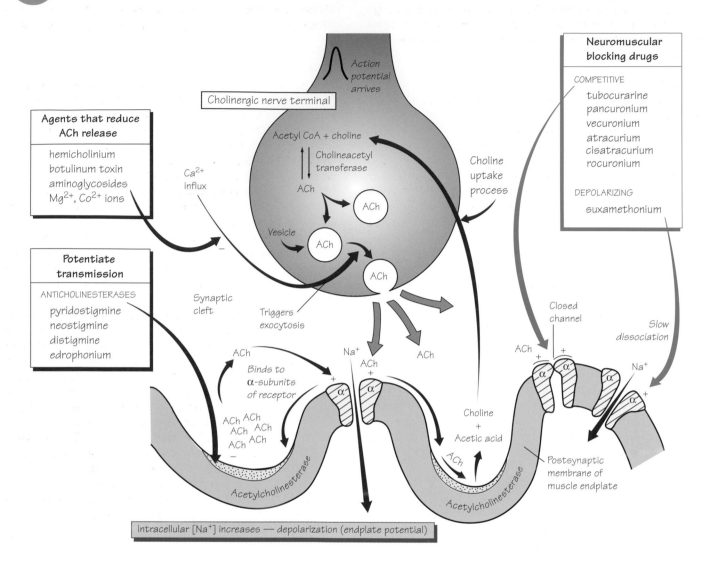

Action potential arrives

Cholinergic nerve terminal

Neuromuscular blocking drugs

COMPETITIVE
tubocurarine
pancuronium
vecuronium
atracurium
cisatracurium
rocuronium

DEPOLARIZING
suxamethonium

Agents that reduce ACh release

hemicholinium
botulinum toxin
aminoglycosides
Mg^{2+}, Co^{2+} ions

Acetyl CoA + choline

Cholineacetyl transferase

ACh

Ca^{2+} influx

Choline uptake process

Vesicle

ACh

Potentiate transmission

ANTICHOLINESTERASES
pyridostigmine
neostigmine
distigmine
edrophonium

Synaptic cleft

Triggers exocytosis

ACh

Closed channel

Slow dissociation

ACh

Binds to α-subunits of receptor

Na^+

ACh

ACh

Na^+

ACh ACh
ACh ACh
ACh ACh

Choline + Acetic acid

Postsynaptic membrane of muscle endplate

Acetylcholinesterase

Acetylcholinesterase

Intracellular $[Na^+]$ increases — depolarization (endplate potential)

Action potentials are conducted along the motor nerves to their terminals (upper figure, ▢), where the depolarization initiates an influx of Ca^{2+} ions and the release of **acetylcholine** (ACh) by a process of **exocytosis** (⇨). The acetylcholine diffuses across the junctional cleft and binds to receptors located on the surface of the muscle fibre membrane at the motor endplate. The reversible combination of acetylcholine and receptors (lower figure, ▨) triggers the opening of cation-selective channels in the endplate membrane, allowing an influx of Na^+ ions and a lesser efflux of K^+ ions. The resulting depolarization, which is called an endplate potential (EPP), depolarizes the adjacent muscle fibre membrane. If large enough, this depolarization results in an action potential and muscle contraction. The acetylcholine released into the synaptic cleft is rapidly hydrolysed by an enzyme, acetylcholinesterase (▦), which is present in the endplate membrane close to the receptors.

Neuromuscular transmission can be increased by **anticholinesterase drugs** (bottom left), which inhibit acetylcholinesterase and slow down the hydrolysis of acetylcholine in the synaptic cleft (see also Chapter 8). *Neostigmine* and *pyridostigmine* are used in the treatment of **myasthenia gravis** and to reverse competitive neuromuscular blockade after

surgery. Overdosage of anticholinesterase results in excess acetylcholine and a depolarization block of motor endplates ('cholinergic crisis'). The muscarinic effects of acetylcholine (see Chapter 7) are also potentiated by anticholinesterases, but are blocked with atropine. Edrophonium has a very short action and is only used to diagnose myasthenia gravis.

Neuromuscular blocking drugs (right) are used by anaesthetists to relax skeletal muscles during surgical operations and to prevent muscle contractions during electroconvulsive therapy (ECT). Most of the clinically useful neuromuscular blocking drugs compete with acetylcholine for the receptor but do not initiate ion channel opening. These **competitive antagonists** reduce the endplate depolarizations produced by acetylcholine to a size that is below the threshold for muscle action potential generation and so cause a flaccid paralysis. **Depolarizing blockers** also act on acetylcholine receptors, but trigger the opening of the ion channels. They are not reversed by anticholinesterases. **Suxamethonium** is the only drug of this type used clinically.

Some agents (top left) act presynaptically and block neuromuscular transmission by preventing the release of acetylcholine.

Acetylcholine

Acetylcholine is synthesized in motor neurone terminals from choline and acetyl coenzyme A (acetyl CoA) by the enzyme choline acetyltransferase. The choline is taken up into the nerve endings from the extracellular fluid by a special choline carrier located in the terminal membrane.

Exocytosis

Acetylcholine is stored in nerve terminals in the cytoplasm and within synaptic vesicles that are anchored to the cytoskeletal network by a protein called synapsin. When an action potential invades the terminal, Ca^{2+} ions enter and activate a protein kinase that phosphorylates synapsin. This results in the detachment of vesicles from their anchorage and fusion with the presynaptic membrane. Several hundred 'packets', or 'quanta', of acetylcholine are released in about a millisecond. This is called quantal release and is very sensitive to the extracellular Ca^{2+} ion concentration. Divalent ions, such as Mg^{2+}, antagonize Ca^{2+} influx and inhibit transmitter release.

Acetylcholine receptors

These can be activated by nicotine and, for this reason, are called **nicotinic receptors**. * The receptor–channel complex is pentameric and is constructed from four different protein subunits ($\alpha\alpha\beta\gamma\epsilon$ in the adult) that span the membrane and are arranged to form a central pore (channel) through which cations (mainly Na^+) flow. Acetylcholine molecules bind to the two α-subunits inducing a conformational change that opens the channel for about 1 ms.

Myasthenia gravis

Myasthenia gravis is an autoimmune disease in which neuromuscular transmission is defective. Circulating heterogeneous immunoglobulin G (IgG) antibodies cause a loss of functional acetylcholine receptors in skeletal muscle. To counteract the loss of, or damage to, receptors, the amount of acetylcholine in the synaptic cleft is increased by the administration of an **anticholinesterase**. Immunological treatment of generalised myasthenia gravis involves the administration of **prednisolone**, usually in combination with **azathioprine** (Chapter 44). Plasmapheresis, in which blood is removed and the cells returned, may improve motor function, presumably by reducing the level of immune complexes. Thymectomy may be curative.

Presynaptic agents

Drugs inhibiting acetylcholine release

Botulinum toxin is produced by *Clostridium botulinum* (an anaerobic bacillus, see Chapter 37). The exotoxin is extraordinarily potent and prevents acetylcholine release by enzymatically cleaving the proteins required for docking of vesicles within the presynaptic membrane. *C. botulinum* is very rarely responsible for serious food poisoning in which the victims exhibit progressive parasympathetic and motor paralysis. **Botulinum toxin type A** is used in the treatment of certain dystonias, such as blepharospasm (spasmodic eye closure) and hemifacial spasm. In these conditions, low doses of toxin are injected into the appropriate muscle to produce paralysis, which persists for about 12 weeks.

* Pentameric nicotinic receptors also occur in autonomic ganglia and the brain. They have variants of the α- and β-subunit and a different pharmacology.

Aminoglycoside antibiotics (e.g. gentamicin) may cause neuromuscular blockade by inhibiting the calcium influx required for exocytosis. This unwanted effect usually occurs only as the result of an interaction with neuromuscular blockers. Myasthenia gravis may be exacerbated.

Competitive neuromuscular blocking drugs

In general, the competitive neuromuscular blocking drugs are bulky, rigid molecules and most have two quaternary N atoms. Neuromuscular blocking drugs are given by intravenous injection and are distributed in the extracellular fluid. They do not cross the blood–brain barrier or the placenta. The choice of a particular drug is often determined by the side-effects produced. These include histamine release, vagal blockade, ganglion blockade and sympathomimetic actions. The onset of action and the duration of action of neuromuscular blocking drugs depend on the dose, but also on other factors (e.g. prior use of suxamethonium, anaesthetic agent used).

Tubocurarine was introduced in 1942 but is no longer used.

Pancuronium is an aminosteroid neuromuscular blocking drug with a relatively long duration of action. It does not block ganglia or cause histamine release. However, it has a dose-related atropine-like effect on the heart that can produce tachycardia.

Vecuronium and atracurium are commonly used agents. Vecuronium has no cardiovascular effects. It depends on hepatic inactivation, and recovery can occur within 20–30 min, making it an attractive drug for short procedures. Atracurium has a duration of action of 15–30 min. It is only stable when kept cold and at low pH. At body pH and temperature it decomposes spontaneously in plasma and therefore does not depend on renal or hepatic function for its elimination. It is the drug of choice in patients with severe renal or hepatic disease. Atracurium may cause histamine release with flushing and hypotension. **Cisatracurium** is an isomer of atracurium. Its main advantage is that it does not cause histamine release and associated cardiovascular effects.

Rocuronium has an intermediate duration of action of about 30 min, but a rapid onset of action (1–2 min) comparable with that of suxamethonium (1–1.5 min). It has minimal cardiovascular effects.

Depolarizing neuromuscular blocking drugs

Suxamethonium (succinylcholine) is used because of its rapid onset and very short duration of action (2–6 min). The drug is normally hydrolysed rapidly by plasma pseudocholinesterase, but a few people inherit an atypical form of the enzyme and, in such individuals, the neuromuscular block may last for hours. Suxamethonium depolarizes the endplate and, because the drug does not dissociate rapidly from the receptors, a prolonged receptor activation is produced. The resulting endplate depolarization initially causes a brief train of muscle action potentials and muscle fibre twitches. Neuromuscular block then occurs as a result of several factors, which include: (i) inactivation of the voltage-sensitive Na^+ channels in the surrounding muscle fibre membrane, so that action potentials are no longer generated; and (ii) transformation of the activated receptors to a 'desensitized' state, unresponsive to acetylcholine. The main disadvantage of suxamethonium is that the initial asynchronous muscle fibre twitches cause damage, which often results in muscle pains the next day. The damage also causes potassium release. Repeated doses of suxamethonium may cause bradycardia in the absence of atropine (a muscarinic effect).

7 Autonomic nervous system

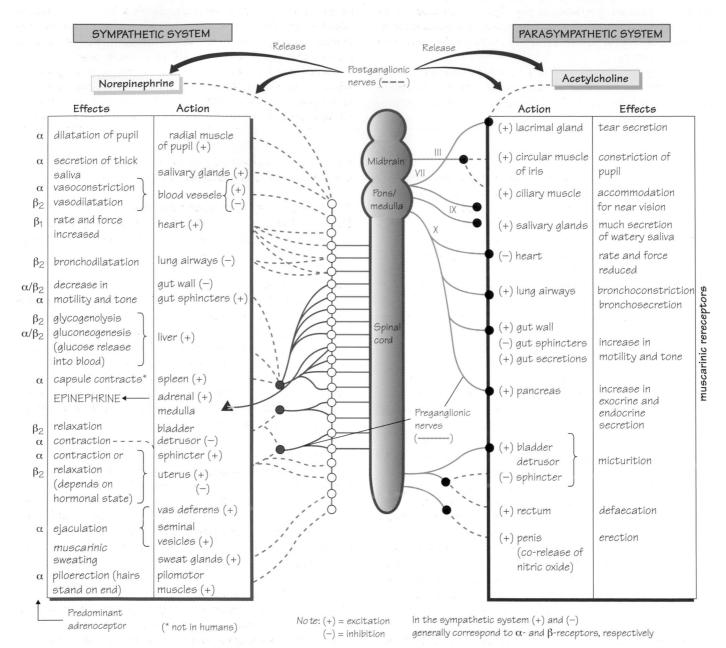

Many systems of the body (e.g. digestion, circulation) are controlled automatically by the autonomic nervous system (and the endocrine system). Control of the autonomic nervous system often involves negative feedback, and there are many afferent (sensory) fibres that carry information to centres in the hypothalamus and medulla. These centres control the outflow of the autonomic nervous system, which is divided on anatomical grounds into two major parts: the **sympathetic system** (left) and the **parasympathetic system** (right). Many organs are innervated by both systems, which in general have opposing actions. The actions of sympathetic (left) and parasympathetic (right) stimulation on different tissues are indicated in the inner columns, and the resulting effects on different organs are shown in the outer columns.

The sympathetic nerves (left, ——) leave the thoracolumbar region of the spinal cord (T1–L3) and synapse either in the **paravertebral**

ganglia (○) or in the **prevertebral ganglia** (●) and plexuses in the abdominal cavity. Postganglionic non-myelinated nerve fibres (left, - - - -) arising from neurones in the ganglia innervate most organs of the body (left).

The transmitter substance released at sympathetic nerve endings is noradrenaline (**norepinephrine**; top left). Inactivation of this transmitter occurs largely by reuptake into the nerve terminals. Some preganglionic sympathetic fibres pass directly to the adrenal medulla (▲), which can release adrenaline (**epinephrine**) into the circulation. Norepinephrine and epinephrine produce their actions on effector organs by acting on α-, β_1- or β_2-**adrenoceptors** (extreme left).

In the parasympathetic system, the preganglionic fibres (right, ——) leave the central nervous system via the cranial nerves (especially III, VII, IX and X) and the third and fourth sacral spinal roots. They often travel much further than sympathetic fibres before synapsing in ganglia (●), which are often in the tissue itself (right).

The nerve endings of the postganglionic parasympathetic fibres (right, - - -) release **acetylcholine** (top right), which produces its actions on the effector organs (right) by activating muscarinic receptors. Acetylcholine released at synapses is inactivated by the enzyme acetylcholinesterase.

All the preganglionic nerve fibres (sympathetic and parasympathetic, ——) are myelinated and release acetylcholine from the nerve terminals; the acetylcholine depolarizes the ganglionic neurones by activating nicotinic receptors.

A small proportion of autonomic nerves release neither acetylcholine nor norepinephrine. For example, the cavernous nerves release nitric oxide (NO) in the penis. This relaxes the smooth muscle of the corpora cavernosa (via cyclic guanosine monophosphate [cGMP], Chapter 16) allowing expansion of the lacunar spaces and erection. **Sildenafil**, used in male sexual dysfunction, inhibits phosphodiesterase type 5 and, by increasing the concentration of cGMP, facilitates erection.

Adrenaline mimics most sympathetic effects, i.e. it is a *sympathomimetic agent* (Chapter 9). Elliot suggested in 1904 that adrenaline was the sympathetic transmitter substance, but Dale pointed out in 1910 that **noradrenaline** mimicked sympathetic nerve stimulation more closely.

Effects of sympathetic stimulation

These are most easily remembered by thinking of changes in the body that are appropriate in the '*fright or flight reaction*'. Note which of the following effects are excitatory and which are inhibitory.

1 Pupillary dilatation (more light reaches the retina).

2 Bronchiolar dilatation (facilitates increased ventilation).

3 Heart rate and force are increased; blood pressure rises (more blood for increased activity of skeletal muscles – running!).

4 Vasoconstriction in skin and viscera and vasodilatation in skeletal muscles (appropriate redistribution of blood to muscles).

5 To provide extra energy, glycogenolysis is stimulated and the blood glucose level increases. The gastrointestinal tract and urinary bladder relax.

Adrenoceptors

These are divided into two main types: *α-receptors* mediate the excitatory effects of sympathomimetic amines, whereas their inhibitory effects are generally mediated by *β-receptors* (exceptions are the smooth muscle of the gut, for which α-stimulation is inhibitory, and the heart, for which β-stimulation is excitatory). Responses mediated by α- and β-receptors can be distinguished by: (i) phentolamine and propranolol, which *selectively* block α- and β-receptors, respectively; and (ii) the relative potencies, on different tissues, of norepinephrine (NE), epinephrine (E) and isoprenaline (I). The order of potency is NE > E > I where excitatory (α) responses are examined, but for inhibitory (β) responses this order is reversed (I >> E > NE).

β-Adrenoceptors are not homogeneous. For example, norepinephrine is an effective stimulant of cardiac β-receptors, but has little or no action on the β-receptors mediating vasodilatation. On the basis of the type of differential sensitivity they exhibit to drugs, β-receptors are divided into two types: β_1 (heart, intestinal smooth muscle) and β_2 (bronchial, vascular and uterine smooth muscle).

α-Adrenoceptors are divided into two classes, originally depending on whether their location is postsynaptic (α_1) or presynaptic (α_2). Stimulation of the presynaptic α_2-receptors by synaptically released norepinephrine reduces further transmitter release (negative feedback). Postsynaptic α_2-receptors occur in a few tissues, e.g. brain, vascular smooth muscle (but mainly α_1).

Acetylcholine

Acetylcholine is the transmitter substance released by the following:

1 All preganglionic autonomic nerves (i.e. both sympathetic and parasympathetic).

2 Postganglionic parasympathetic nerves.

3 Some postganglionic sympathetic nerves (i.e. thermoregulatory sweat glands and skeletal muscle vasodilator fibres).

4 Nerve to the adrenal medulla.

5 Somatic motor nerves to skeletal muscle endplates (Chapter 6).

6 Some neurones in the central nervous system (Chapter 22).

Acetylcholine receptors (cholinoceptors)

These are divided into nicotinic and muscarinic subtypes (originally determined by measuring the sensitivity of various tissues to the drugs nicotine and muscarine, respectively).

Muscarinic receptors

Acetylcholine released at the nerve terminals of postganglionic parasympathetic fibres acts on muscarinic receptors and can be blocked selectively by atropine. Five subtypes of muscarinic receptor exist, three of which have been well characterized: M_1, M_2 and M_3. M_1-receptors occur in the brain and gastric parietal cells, M_2-receptors in the heart and M_3-receptors in smooth muscle and glands. Except for **pirenzepine**, which selectively blocks M_1-receptors (Chapter 12), clinically useful muscarinic agonists and antagonists show little or no selectivity for the different subtypes of muscarinic receptor.

Nicotinic receptors

These occur in autonomic ganglia and in the adrenal medulla, where the effects of acetylcholine (or nicotine) can be blocked selectively with hexamethonium. The nicotinic receptors at the skeletal muscle neuromuscular junction are not blocked by hexamethonium, but are blocked by tubocurarine. Thus, receptors at ganglia and neuromuscular junctions are different, although both types are stimulated by nicotine and therefore called nicotinic.

Actions of acetylcholine

Muscarinic effects are mainly parasympathomimetic (except sweating and vasodilatation), and in general are the opposite of those caused by sympathetic stimulation. Muscarinic effects include: constriction of the pupil, accommodation for near vision (Chapter 10), profuse watery salivation, bronchiolar constriction, bronchosecretion, hypotension (as a result of bradycardia and vasodilatation), an increase in gastrointestinal motility and secretion, contraction of the urinary bladder and sweating.

Nicotinic effects include stimulation of all autonomic ganglia. However, the action of acetylcholine on ganglia is relatively weak compared with its effect on muscarinic receptors, and so parasympathetic effects predominate. The nicotinic actions of acetylcholine on the sympathetic system can be demonstrated, for example, on cat blood pressure, by blocking its muscarinic actions with atropine. High intravenous doses of acetylcholine then cause a rise in blood pressure, because stimulation of the sympathetic ganglia and adrenal medulla now results in vasoconstriction and tachycardia.

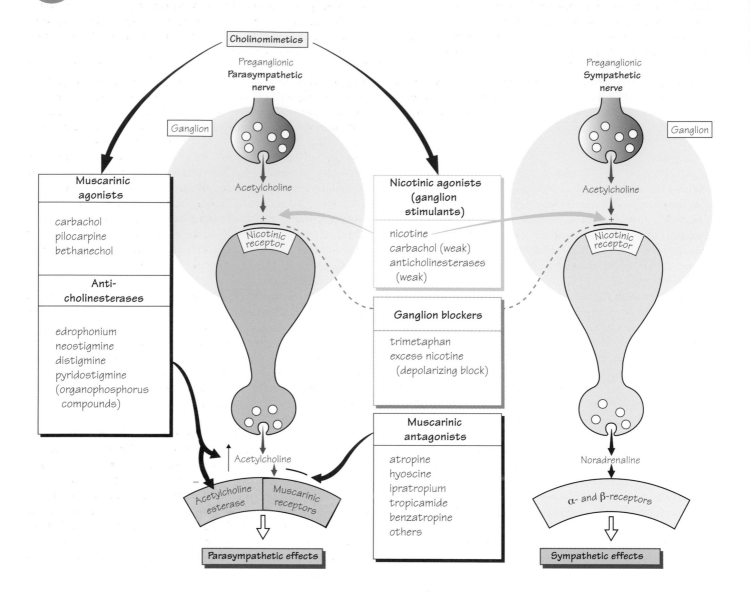

Acetylcholine released from the terminals of postganglionic parasympathetic nerves (left, ▨) produces its actions on various effector organs by activating **muscarinic receptors** (▨). The effects of acetylcholine are usually excitatory, but an important exception is the heart, which receives inhibitory cholinergic fibres from the vagus (Chapter 17). Drugs that mimic the effects of acetylcholine are called **cholinomimetics** and can be divided into two groups:
• drugs that act directly on receptors (**nicotinic** and **muscarinic agonists**); and
• **anticholinesterases**, which inhibit acetylcholinesterase, and so act indirectly by allowing acetylcholine to accumulate in the synapse and produce its effects.

Muscarinic agonists (top left) have few uses, but **pilocarpine** and **carbachol** (as eyedrops) are sometimes used to reduce intraocular pressure in patients with glaucoma (Chapter 10). **Bethanechol** was used to stimulate the bladder in urinary retention, but it has been superseded by catheterization.

Anticholinesterases (bottom left) have relatively little effect at ganglia and are used mainly for their nicotinic effects on the neuromuscular junction. They are used in the treatment of myasthenia gravis and to reverse the effects of competitive muscle relaxants used during surgery (Chapter 6).

Muscarinic antagonists (bottom middle) block the effects of acetylcholine released from postganglionic parasympathetic nerve terminals. Their effects can, in general, be worked out by examination of the figure in Chapter 7. However, parasympathetic effector organs vary in their sensitivity to the blocking effect of antagonists. Secretions of the salivary, bronchial and sweat glands are most sensitive to blockade. Higher doses of antagonist dilate the pupils, paralyse accommodation and produce tachycardia by blocking vagal tone in the heart. Still higher doses inhibit parasympathetic control of the gastrointestinal tract and bladder. Gastric acid secretion is most resistant to blockade (Chapter 12).

Atropine, **hyoscine** (scopolamine) or other antagonists are used:
1 in anaesthesia to block vagal slowing of the heart and to inhibit bronchial secretion;

2 to reduce intestinal spasm in, for example, irritable bowel syndrome (Chapter 13);

3 in Parkinson's disease (e.g. benzatropine, Chapter 26);

4 to prevent motion sickness (hyoscine, Chapter 30);

5 to dilate the pupil for ophthalmological examination (e.g. tropicamide) or to paralyse the ciliary muscle (Chapter 10); and

6 as a bronchodilator in asthma (ipratropium, Chapter 11).

Transmission at autonomic ganglia ( ) can be stimulated by nicotinic agonists (top middle) or blocked by drugs that act specifically on the ganglionic neurone nicotinic receptor/ionophore (middle). Nicotinic agonists are of no clinical use and ganglion blocking drugs, eg hexamethonium, are only of historical interest.

Cholinergic nerve terminals in the autonomic nervous system synthesize, store and release acetylcholine in essentially the same way as at the neuromuscular junction (Chapter 6). Acetylcholinesterase is bound to both the pre- and postsynaptic membranes.

Cholinomimetics

Ganglion stimulants

These have widespread actions because they stimulate nicotinic receptors on both parasympathetic and sympathetic ganglionic neurones. Sympathetic effects include vasoconstriction, tachycardia and hypertension. Parasympathetic effects include increased motility of the gut and increased salivary and bronchial secretion. They have no clinical uses.

Muscarinic agonists

These directly activate muscarinic receptors, usually producing excitatory effects. An important exception is the heart, where activation of the predominantly M_2-receptors has inhibitory effects on the rate and force of (atrial) contraction. The M_2-receptors are negatively coupled by a G-protein (G_1) to adenylyl cyclase, which explains the negative inotropic effect of acetylcholine. Subunits $(\beta\gamma)$ of G_1 directly increase K^+ conductances in the heart, causing hyperpolarization and bradycardia (Chapter 17). Acetylcholine stimulates glandular secretion and causes contraction of smooth muscle by activating M_3-receptors, which are coupled to the formation of inositol-1,4,5-trisphosphate $(InsP_3)$ and diacylglycerol (Chapter 1). $InsP_3$ increases cytosolic Ca^{2+}, thus triggering muscle contraction or glandular secretion. An intravenous injection of acetylcholine causes vasodilatation indirectly by releasing nitric oxide (NO) from vascular endothelial cells (Chapter 16). However, most blood vessels have no parasympathetic innervation and so the physiological function of vascular muscarinic receptors is uncertain.

Choline esters

Carbachol and **bethanechol** are quaternary compounds that do not penetrate the blood–brain barrier. Their actions are much more prolonged than those of acetylcholine, because they are not hydrolysed by cholinesterase.

Pilocarpine possesses a tertiary N atom, which confers increased lipid solubility. This enables the drug to penetrate the cornea readily when applied locally, and enter the brain when given systemically.

Anticholinesterases

These are indirectly acting cholinomimetics. The commonly used anticholinesterase drugs are quaternary compounds that do not pass the blood–brain barrier and have negligible central effects. They are poorly absorbed orally. **Physostigmine** (eserine) is much more lipid soluble. It is well absorbed after oral or local administration (e.g. as eyedrops) and passes into the brain.

Mechanism of action

Initially, acetylcholine binds to the active site of the esterase and is hydrolysed, producing free choline and acetylated enzyme. In a second step, the covalent acetyl–enzyme bond is split with the addition of water. **Edrophonium** is the main example of a reversible anticholinesterase. It binds by electrostatic forces to the active site of the enzyme. It does not form covalent bonds with the enzyme and so is very short acting (2–10 min). The carbamate esters (e.g. **neostigmine**, **pyridostigmine**) undergo the same two-step process as acetylcholine, except that the breakdown of the carbamylated enzyme is much slower (30 min to 6 h). Organophosphorus agents (e.g. **ecothiopate**) result in a phosphorylated enzyme active site. The covalent phosphorus–enzyme bond is very stable and the enzyme is inactivated for hundreds of hours. For this reason, the organophosphorus compounds are referred to as irreversible anticholinesterases. They are extremely toxic and are used as insecticides (parathion, malathion) and chemical warfare agents (e.g. sarin).

The **effects of anticholinesterases** are generally similar to those produced by the directly acting muscarinic agonists, but, in addition, transmission at the neuromuscular junction is potentiated. The cholinesterase inhibitors produce less vasodilatation than the directly acting agonists because they can only act on the (few) vessels possessing cholinergic innervation. Also, stimulation of sympathetic ganglia may oppose the vasodilator effects of the drug. Only large toxic doses of anticholinesterase produce marked bradycardia and hypotension.

Toxic doses initially cause signs of extreme muscarinic stimulation: miosis, salivation, sweating, bronchial constriction, bronchosecretion, vomiting and diarrhoea. Excessive stimulation of nicotinic receptors may cause depolarizing neuromuscular blockade. If the drug is lipid soluble (e.g. organophosphorus compounds, except ecothiopate), convulsions, coma and respiratory arrest may occur. Strong nucleophiles (e.g. **pralidoxime**) can split the phosphorus–enzyme bond initially formed by organophosphorus compounds and 'regenerate' the enzyme. Later, this becomes impossible because a process of 'ageing' strengthens the phosphorus–enzyme bond.

Cholinergic receptor antagonists

Ganglion blockers

These cause hypotension, mydriasis, dry mouth, anhidrosis, constipation, urinary retention and impotence. **Trimetaphan** is given as an intravenous infusion to produce controlled hypotension during certain surgical procedures.

Muscarinic antagonists (antimuscarinics)

Atropine occurs in deadly nightshade (*Atropa belladonna*). It is a weak central stimulant, especially on the vagal nucleus, and low doses often cause bradycardia. Higher doses cause tachycardia. **Hyoscine** (scopolamine) is more sedative than atropine and often produces drowsiness and amnesia. Toxic doses of both drugs cause excitement, agitation, hallucination and coma. The effects of muscarinic antagonists can be worked out by studying the figure in Chapter 7. The student should understand why these drugs produce dilated pupils, blurred vision, dry mouth, constipation and difficulty with micturition.

9 Drugs acting on the sympathetic system

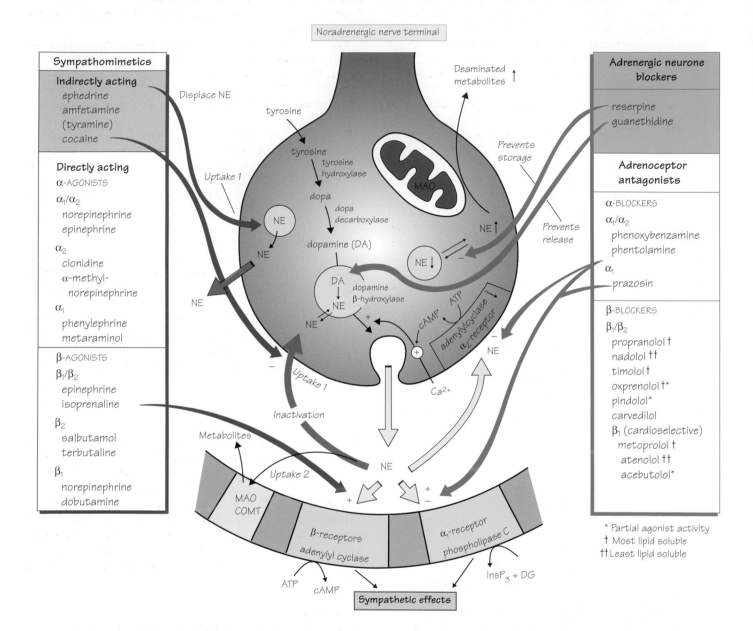

Sympathomimetics

Indirectly acting
- ephedrine
- amfetamine
- (tyramine)
- cocaine

Directly acting

α-AGONISTS

α₁/α₂
- norepinephrine
- epinephrine

α₂
- clonidine
- α-methyl-norepinephrine

α₁
- phenylephrine
- metaraminol

β-AGONISTS

β₁/β₂
- epinephrine
- isoprenaline

β₂
- salbutamol
- terbutaline

β₁
- norepinephrine
- dobutamine

Adrenergic neurone blockers
- reserpine
- guanethidine

Adrenoceptor antagonists

α-BLOCKERS

α₁/α₂
- phenoxybenzamine
- phentolamine

α₁
- prazosin

β-BLOCKERS

β₁/β₂
- propranolol †
- nadolol ††
- timolol †
- oxprenolol †*
- pindolol*
- carvedilol

β₁ (cardioselective)
- metoprolol †
- atenolol ††
- acebutolol*

* Partial agonist activity
† Most lipid soluble
†† Least lipid soluble

The sympathetic nervous system is important in regulating organs such as the heart and peripheral vasculature (Chapters 15 and 18). The transmitter released from sympathetic nerve endings is **norepinephrine (NE)** (noradrenaline, ⇨) but, in response to some forms of stress, **epinephrine** (adrenaline) is also released from the adrenal medulla. These catecholamines are inactivated mainly by **reuptake** (➡).

Sympathomimetics (left) are drugs that partially or completely mimic the actions of norepinephrine and epinephrine. They act either **directly** on α- and/or β-adrenoceptors (left, open column) or **indirectly** on the presynaptic terminals (top left, shaded blue), usually by causing the release of norepinephrine (⇨). The effects of adrenoceptor stimulation can be seen in the figure in Chapter 7.

β₂-Adrenoceptor agonists cause bronchial dilatation and are used in the treatment of asthma (Chapter 11). They are also used to relax uterine muscle in an attempt to prevent preterm labour. **β₁-Adrenoceptor agonists** (dobutamine) are sometimes used to stimulate the force of heart contraction in severe low-output heart failure (Chapter 18). **α₁-Agonists** (e.g. **phenylephrine**) are used as mydriatics (Chapter 10) and in many popular decongestant preparations. **α₂-Agonists**, notably **clonidine** and **methyldopa** (which acts after its conversion to α-methylnorepinephrine, a false transmitter), are centrally acting hypotensive drugs (Chapter 15).

Sympathomimetic amines that act mainly by causing **norepinephrine release** (e.g. **amfetamine**) have the α₁/α₂ selectivity of norepinephrine. **Ephedrine**, in addition to causing norepinephrine release, also has a direct action. Its effects resemble those of epinephrine, but last much longer. Ephedrine is a mild central stimulant, but amfetamine, which enters the brain more readily, has a much greater stimulant effect on mood and alertness and a depressant effect on appetite. Amfetamine and similar drugs have a high abuse potential and are rarely used (Chapter 31).

β-Adrenoceptor antagonists (**β-blockers**) (bottom right) are important drugs in the treatment of hypertension (Chapter 15), angina (Chapter 16), cardiac arrhythmias (Chapter 17), heart failure (Chapter 18) and glaucoma (Chapter 10). **α-Adrenoceptor antagonists** (**α-blockers**) (middle right) have limited clinical applications. **Prazosin**, a selective α_1-antagonist, is sometimes used in the treatment of hypertension. **Phenoxybenzamine**, an irreversible antagonist, is used to block the α-effects of the large amounts of catecholamines released from tumours of the adrenal medulla (phaeochromocytoma). Phentolamine, a short-acting drug, is used during surgery of phaeochromocytoma.

Adrenergic neurone-blocking drugs (top right, shaded) either deplete the nerve terminals of norepinephrine (**reserpine**) or prevent its release. They were used as hypotensive agents (Chapter 15).

Reuptake of norepinephrine by a high-affinity transport system (Uptake 1) in the nerve terminals 'recaptures' most of the transmitter and is the main method of terminating its effects. A similar (extraneuronal) transport system (Uptake 2) exists in the tissues but is less selective and less easily saturated.

Monoamine oxidase (**MAO**) and **catechol-*O*-methyltransferase** (**COMT**) are widely distributed enzymes that catabolize catecholamines. Inhibition of MAO and COMT has little potentiating effect on responses to sympathetic nerve stimulation or injected catecholamines (norepinephrine, epinephrine) because they are largely inactivated by reuptake.

α_1-**Adrenoceptors** are postsynaptic. Their activation in several tissues (e.g. smooth muscle, salivary glands) causes an increase in inositol-1,4,5-trisphosphate and subsequently cytosolic calcium (Chapter 1), which triggers vasoconstriction or glandular secretion.

α_2-**Adrenoceptors** occur on noradrenergic nerve terminals. Their activation by norepinephrine inhibits adenylyl cyclase. The consequent fall in cyclic adenosine monophosphate (cAMP) closes Ca^{2+} channels and diminishes further transmitter release.

β-Adrenoceptor activation results in stimulation of adenylyl cyclase, increasing the conversion of adenosine triphosphate (ATP) to cAMP. The cAMP acts as a 'second messenger', coupling receptor activation to response.

Sympathomimetics

Indirectly acting sympathomimetics
Indirectly acting sympathomimetics resemble the structure of norepinephrine closely enough to be transported by Uptake 1 into nerve terminals where they displace vesicular norepinephrine into the cytoplasm. Some of the norepinephrine is metabolized by MAO, but the remainder is released by carrier-mediated transport to activate adrenoceptors.

Amfetamines are resistant to MAO. Their peripheral actions (e.g. tachycardia, hypertension) and central stimulant actions are mainly caused by catecholamine release. **Dexamfetamine** and **methylphenidate** are sometimes used in hyperkinetic children. Dexamfetamine and **modafinil** may be beneficial in narcolepsy. Dependence on amfetamine-like drugs is common (Chapter 31).

Cocaine, in addition to being a local anaesthetic (Chapter 5), is a sympathomimetic because it inhibits the reuptake of norepinephrine by nerve terminals. It has an intense central stimulant effect that has made it a popular drug of abuse (Chapter 31).

Directly acting sympathomimetics
The effect of sympathomimetic drugs in humans depends on their receptor specificity (α and/or β) and on the compensatory reflexes they evoke.

Epinephrine and **norepinephrine** are destroyed in the gut and are short lasting when injected because of uptake and metabolism. Epinephrine increases the blood pressure by stimulating the rate and force of the heart beat (β_1-effects). Stimulation of vascular α-receptors causes vasoconstriction (viscera, skin), but β_2-stimulation causes vasodilatation (skeletal muscle) and the total peripheral resistance may actually decrease.

Norepinephrine has little or no effect on the vascular β_2-receptors, and so the α-mediated vasoconstriction is unopposed. The resulting rise in blood pressure reflexively slows the heart, usually overcoming the direct β_1-stimulant action on the heart rate.

Epinephrine by injection has an important use in the treatment of *anaphylactic shock* (Chapter 11).

β-Receptor-selective drugs
Isoprenaline stimulates all β-receptors, increasing the rate and force of the heart beat and causing vasodilatation. These effects result in a fall in diastolic and mean arterial pressure with little change in systolic pressure.

β_2-**Adrenoceptor agonists** are relatively selective drugs that produce bronchodilatation at doses that cause minimal effects on the heart. They are resistant to MAO and are probably not taken up into neurones. Their main use is in the treatment of asthma (Chapter 11).

Adrenoceptor antagonists

α-Blockers
α-Blockers reduce arteriolar and venous tone, causing a fall in peripheral resistance and hypotension (Chapter 15). They reverse the pressor effects of epinephrine, because the β_2-mediated vasodilator effects of the latter are unopposed by α-mediated vasoconstriction and the peripheral resistance falls (epinephrine reversal). α-Blockers cause a reflex tachycardia, which is greater with non-selective drugs that also block α_2-presynaptic receptors in the heart, because the augmented release of norepinephrine stimulates further the cardiac β-receptors. **Prazosin**, a selective α_1-antagonist, causes relatively little tachycardia.

β-Blockers
β-Blockers vary in their *lipid solubility* and *cardioselectivity*. However, they all block β_1-receptors and are equally effective in reducing blood pressure and preventing angina. The more lipid-soluble drugs are more rapidly absorbed from the gut, undergo more first-pass hepatic metabolism and are more rapidly eliminated. They are also more likely to enter the brain and cause central effects (e.g. bad dreams). *Cardioselectivity* is only relative and diminishes with higher doses. Nevertheless, selective β_1-blockade seems to produce less peripheral vasoconstriction (cold hands and feet) and does not reduce the response to exercise-induced hypoglycaemia (stimulation of gluconeogenesis in the liver is mediated by β_2-receptors). Cardioselective drugs may have sufficient β_2-activity to precipitate severe bronchospasm in patients with asthma, and such patients should avoid β-blockers. Some β-blockers possess *intrinsic sympathomimetic activity* (i.e. are partial agonists, Chapter 2). The clinical importance of this is debatable, but see Chapter 16.

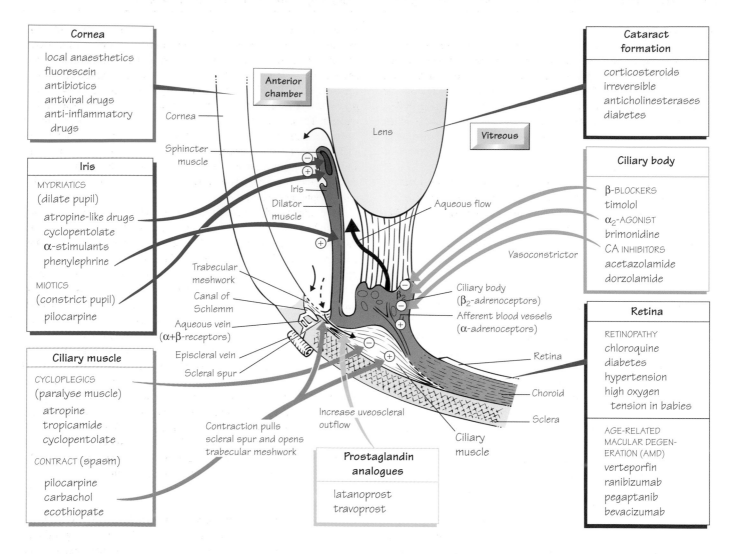

Cornea

local anaesthetics
fluorescein
antibiotics
antiviral drugs
anti-inflammatory
 drugs

Iris

MYDRIATICS
(dilate pupil)
 atropine-like drugs
 cyclopentolate
 α-stimulants
 phenylephrine

MIOTICS
(constrict pupil)
 pilocarpine

Ciliary muscle

CYCLOPLEGICS
(paralyse muscle)
 atropine
 tropicamide
 cyclopentolate

CONTRACT (spasm)
 pilocarpine
 carbachol
 ecothiopate

**Cataract
formation**

corticosteroids
irreversible
anticholinesterases
diabetes

Ciliary body

β-BLOCKERS
 timolol
α₂-AGONIST
 brimonidine
CA INHIBITORS
 acetazolamide
 dorzolamide

Retina

RETINOPATHY
 chloroquine
 diabetes
 hypertension
 high oxygen
  tension in babies

AGE-RELATED
MACULAR DEGEN-
ERATION (AMD)
 verteporfin
 ranibizumab
 pegaptanib
 bevacizumab

**Prostaglandin
analogues**

 latanoprost
 travoprost

The eye is an inflated spherical shell, its outer layer being the tough, collagen-rich sclera. The normal **intraocular pressure** (IOP) is about 15 mmHg. It is maintained by a balance of aqueous humour formation by the *ciliary body* (➡) and outflow through the *trabecular mesh-work* into the canal of Schlemm (↶) or the uveoscleral pathway (▼--). In open-angle **glaucoma**, pathological changes in the trabecular meshwork decrease the outflow of aqueous. Because the resulting elevated IOP will eventually damage the optic nerve, the pressure is reduced, usually with topical drugs. This can be achieved either by increasing aqueous outflow with **prostaglandin analogues** (bottom centre) or, rarely, with **muscarinic agonists**, such as **pilocarpine** (bottom left), or by reducing aqueous formation with a variety of drugs (middle right), but especially **timolol**, a β-blocker.

At the front of the eye, the sclera runs into the **cornea** (top left), whose transparency is obtained by alignment of the collagen fibres. Many superficial manipulations, such as tonometry (measurement of the IOP) and the removal of corneal foreign bodies, require the instillation of a *local anaesthetic*. **Fluorescein** is commonly instilled into the eye to reveal damaged areas of corneal epithelium, which are stained bright green by the dye. **Inflammation** of the cornea resulting from allergy or chemical burns is treated with topical anti-inflammatory drugs (Chapter 33). Infections are not treated with anti-inflammatory agents, except together with an effective chemotherapeutic agent, because anti-inflammatory drugs reduce resistance to invading microorganisms.

The **iris** (middle left) possesses a sphincter muscle, which receives parasympathetic nerves, and a dilator muscle, which is innervated by sympathetic fibres. Thus, muscarinic antagonists and α-adrenoceptor agonists *dilate* the pupil (**mydriasis**), whereas muscarinic agonists and α-adrenoceptor antagonists *constrict* the pupil (**miosis**).

Contraction of the parasympathetically innervated **ciliary muscle** (bottom left) allows the lens to become thicker and accommodation for near vision occurs. Thus, muscarinic antagonists *paralyse* the ciliary muscle (**cycloplegia**) and prevent accommodation for near vision, whereas agonists cause accommodation and a loss of far vision.

The **lens** (middle top) provides the adjustable part of the eye's refractive power. Opacity of the lens is called a cataract. Some drugs, notably corticosteroids, may cause cataracts.

The **retina** is a part of the central nervous system, but it seems little affected by drugs, probably because of the effective blood–retinal barrier. **Verteporfin** and inhibitors of Vascular endothelial growth factor (bottom right) are used to treat age-related macular degeneration (AMD). The retina may occasionally be damaged by drugs (e.g. bottom right) or by high oxygen tension in newborn babies.

Ciliary body

The processes of the ciliary body are highly vascularized and are the sites of aqueous humour formation. The ciliary epithelial cells, which contain adenosine triphosphatase (ATPase) and carbonic anhydrase, absorb Na^+ selectively from the stroma and transport it into the intercellular clefts, which open only on the aqueous humour side. The hyperosmolality in the clefts causes water flow from the stroma, producing a continuous flow of aqueous.

Trabecular meshwork

The aqueous humour circulates through the pupil and is drained into the canal of Schlemm, which is a circular gutter within the surface of the sclera at the limbus. The sieve-like trabecular meshwork is the roof of the gutter, through which the aqueous must pass before it is eventually drained away into the episcleral veins. Some aqueous drains through the uveoscleral pathway.

Glaucoma

This is a group of ocular diseases with the common features of abnormally high IOP and ultimate loss of vision if untreated. It occurs in about 1% of people over 40 years of age. Viewed through an ophthalmoscope, the optic disc appears depressed (cupping) because of the loss of nerve fibres. The mechanism by which the nerve fibres are destroyed in glaucoma is unclear, but may involve mechanical factors and/or local ischaemia. Open-angle (chronic simple) glaucoma is the most common form of the disease. At present, lowering the IOP is the only treatment for open-angle glaucoma. Generally, the aim is to use topical drugs or, if they fail, surgery to reduce the IOP by 20–50% of the initial pressure.

In closed-angle glaucoma, the angle between the cornea and the iris is abnormally small. Occasionally, the angle closes completely, preventing aqueous outflow, and the IOP quickly rises. Because permanent damage to the retina can occur during these attacks, the pressure must be reduced as quickly as possible by *intensive instillation of pilocarpine* eyedrops combined, if necessary, with intravenous *acetazolamide* and intravenous *hypertonic mannitol* (an osmotic agent) to remove water.

Drugs that reduce IOP by increasing outflow

Latanoprost is a prodrug of prostaglandin F_2 (PGF_2) that passes through the cornea and reduces the IOP by increasing the uveoscleral outflow of aqueous. The mechanism is thought to involve the activation of matrix metalloproteinases leading to a reduction in outflow resistance. Latanoprost is very effective and has reduced the number of patients requiring surgery. It has minimal systemic side-effects and is widely used.

Pilocarpine reduces the IOP by contracting the ciliary muscle. This pulls the scleral spur and results in the trabecular meshwork being stretched and separated. The fluid pathways are opened up and aqueous outflow is increased. All parasympathomimetics cause miosis, resulting in poor night vision and complaints of 'dimming of vision'. Ciliary muscle spasm that increases near-sightedness causing blurred vision is not usually a problem in the age group that develops glaucoma, but can cause headache and browache.

Drugs that reduce IOP by decreasing aqueous secretion

β-Blockers (e.g. **timolol**) block $β_2$-adrenoceptors on the ciliary processes and so reduce aqueous secretion. In addition, they may block β-receptors in the afferent blood vessels supplying the ciliary processes. The resulting vasoconstriction produces reduced ultrafiltration and aqueous formation. Drugs given as eyedrops can be absorbed through the nasal mucosa and produce systemic effects. Thus, β-blockers may provoke bronchospasm in asthmatics or bradycardia in susceptible patients. Therefore, β-blockers (even selective $β_1$-antagonists) should be avoided in patients with asthma, heart failure, heart block or bradycardia.

Brimonidine and **apraclonidine** are $α_2$-adrenoceptor agonists. They decrease aqueous formation by stimulating $α_2$-receptors on the adrenergic nerve terminals innervating the ciliary body (thus reducing norepinephrine release).

Carbonic anhydrase inhibitors. Acetazolamide acts on the ciliary body and prevents bicarbonate synthesis. This leads to a fall in sodium transport and aqueous formation because bicarbonate and sodium transport are linked (Chapter 14). Acetazolamide is given orally or intravenously, but is too toxic for long-term use. **Dorzolamide** is a topically active inhibitor of carbonic anhydrase (CA-2). It can be used alone in patients in whom β-blockers are contraindicated. It is a sulphonamide and systemic side-effects may occur, e.g. skin rashes, bronchospasm.

Laser trabecular surgery may be used as an alternative to drugs in glaucoma. Under local anaesthesia, the surgeon uses an argon or diode laser to place about 100 evenly spaced lesions on the inner surface of the trabecular meshwork. The laser 'burns' cause localized shrinkage, which exerts tension on the adjacent, untreated tissue, opening spaces in the meshwork and allowing increased aqueous drainage. In closed-angle glaucoma, a yttrium aluminium garnet (YAG) laser may be used to make a hole at the periphery of the iris. This prevents the forward movement of the iris that precipitates acute glaucoma and is usually caused by a partial block of aqueous flow through the pupil.

Mydriatics

Mydriasis (dilatation of the pupil) is required for ophthalmoscopy. The drops most commonly used are the relatively short-acting antimuscarinics **tropicamide** and **cyclopentolate**, which produce both mydriasis and cycloplegia. The α-adrenoceptor stimulant **phenylephrine** may be used to produce mydriasis without affecting the pupillary light reflex or accommodation. Mydriasis may precipitate acute closed-angle glaucoma in susceptible patients, who are usually aged over 60 years.

Age-related macular degeneration

Age-related macular degeneration affects older people and is the most common cause of blindness in the UK. In most patients central retinal cells slowly deteriorate, but in 10% of patients, new fragile blood vessels form under the retina and leak fluid and blood. In this neovascular (wet) form of AMD loss of vision can occur in a few months. The first treatment for wet AMD was photodynamic therapy in which **verteporfin**, a light-sensitive dye, is given intravenously and is taken up by the vascular endothelium. A laser is then applied to the lesion and this activates the dye, releasing toxic free radicals that destroy the new vessels (photodynamic therapy). More recently, neovascular AMD has been treated with the intravitreal injection of ranibizumab, pegaptanib and bevacizumab. These new drugs are antibodies that bind to and inhibit vascular endothelial growth factor (VEGF) in the retina, thereby slowing down the progression of AMD.

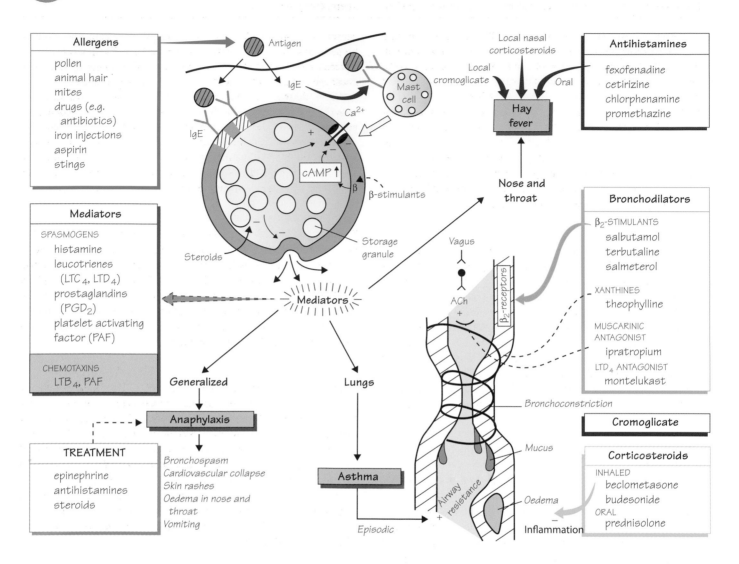

Asthma, hay fever and anaphylaxis (dark red shaded boxes) are caused by the same basic processes: IgE antibody attaches to mast cells (top left) and, on renewed exposure to the same antigen (⊘), degranulation of the mast cells occurs with the production and release of **mediators** (middle left). If the release of mediators is localized, hay fever (top right) or asthma (bottom right) result, but a massive general release causes anaphylaxis, which is a rare but life-threatening reaction to bee stings and penicillin or other drugs. Antigens that can trigger these reactions are called **allergens** (top left).

Bronchial asthma is an inflammatory disease in which the calibre of the airways is chronically narrowed by oedema and is unstable. During an attack the patient suffers from wheezing and difficulty in breathing as a result of bronchospasm, mucosal oedema and mucus formation (bottom right). Eventually the chronic inflammation causes irreversible changes to the airways (bottom right). When the acute attack has an allergic basis, the term *extrinsic asthma* is often used. When there is no obvious allergic basis for the disease, it is called *intrinsic asthma*.

In **mild to moderate asthma**, the first-line drugs are short-acting β_2-adrenoceptor agonists (**β_2-stimulants**, middle right) inhaled from

pressurized containers when required. If β-agonists are required more than once a day, then regular administration of **inhaled steroid** is added (bottom right). In more severe asthma, short-acting β-agonists and inhaled steroids are retained with the addition of a regular inhaled long-acting β-stimulant (e.g. **salmeterol**). If necessary, a high-dose inhaled steroid is tried with salmeterol, together with oral sustained-release **theophylline**, or a modified-release oral β_2-agonist, or a leucotriene receptor antagonist (e.g. **montelukast**; this reduces the bronchoconstrictor and inflammatory effects of leucotriene D_4 [LTD_4]). Some patients are controlled only by oral steroids (usually **prednisolone**, Chapter 33).

Acute severe attacks of asthma (status asthmaticus) that are not controlled by the patient's usual drugs are potentially fatal and must be dealt with as an emergency, requiring hospital admission.

Anaphylaxis (bottom left) requires prompt treatment with **epinephrine** (adrenaline) (Chapter 9), given by intramuscular injection, which is repeated every 5 min until the blood pressure and pulse improve. Oxygen is administered (if available) and **chlorphenamine** (an antihistamine) given intravenously after the epinephrine is useful.

In severe or recurrent anaphylaxis, intravenous or intramuscular **hydrocortisone** is given.

Hay fever is most commonly caused by allergy to grass pollen.

Antihistamines control some symptoms, and nasal corticosteroids are very effective. **Cromoglicate** eyedrops may be a valuable adjunct in allergic conjunctivitis.

IgE is the major class of reaginic antibody. In allergic patients, specific antibody levels may be increased to 100 times greater than normal. Binding of the F_c portion of the antibody to receptors on mast cells, followed by cross-linking of adjacent molecules by antigen, triggers degranulation by a mechanism involving Ca^{2+} influx.

Mast cells contain the body stores of histamine and occur in almost all tissues. Within the mast cells, histamine is bound with heparin in cytoplasmic granules. Histamine release normally involves an influx of Ca^{2+} ions and, because the permeability of the cell membrane to Ca^{2+} ions is reduced when intracellular cyclic adenosine monophosphate (cAMP) levels are raised, drugs that stimulate cAMP synthesis (β_2-adrenoceptor agonists) reduce histamine release.

Mediators

The initial phase of an asthma attack is brought about mainly by spasm of the bronchial smooth muscle caused by the release of **spasmogens** (middle left) from mast cells. In many asthmatics, a second delayed phase results from the release of chemotaxins (centre left, shaded blue) that attract inflammatory cells, especially eosinophils. These inflammatory processes cause *vasodilatation*, *oedema*, *mucus secretion* and *bronchospasm* and are at first reversible. However, permanent damage to the bronchial epithelium and smooth muscle hypertrophy eventually lead to irreversible airway obstruction. This damage seems to be caused mainly by substances released from the eosinophil granules (especially eosinophil major basic protein and granule peroxidase).

Bronchodilators

β-Adrenoceptor stimulants

The airway smooth muscle has few adrenergic nerve fibres but many β_2-receptors, stimulation of which causes bronchodilatation. Activation of β_2-adrenoceptors relaxes smooth muscle by increasing intracellular cAMP, which activates a protein kinase (see nitrates, Chapter 16). This inhibits muscle contraction by phosphorylating and inhibiting myosin-light-chain kinase. β_2-Agonists such as **salbutamol** are usually given by inhalation. They are not specific, but β_1-effects (cardiac stimulation) are not usually seen at doses that cause bronchodilatation. Adverse effects include fine tremor, nervous tension and tachycardia, but these are not usually troublesome when the drug is given by inhalation. Oral administration is usually restricted to children and other patients who cannot use an aerosol preparation. **Salmeterol** is much longer lasting than salbutamol. In contrast to short-acting β_2-agonists, regular treatment with inhaled salmeterol has beneficial effects in asthmatics.

Ipratropium is a muscarinic antagonist and a moderately effective bronchodilator, presumably because it reduces reflex vagal bronchoconstriction that results from histamine stimulation of sensory (irritant) receptors in the airways. Ipratropium given by inhalation rarely causes atropine-like side-effects.

Xanthines

Theophylline may benefit children who cannot use inhalants, and adults with predominantly nocturnal symptoms. Theophylline often causes adverse effects, even oral sustained-release theophylline preparations that are effective for up to 12 h. Even when plasma concentrations are in the therapeutic range ($10–20$ mg L^{-1}), nausea, headache, insomnia and abdominal discomfort are common.

Above 25 mg L^{-1}, toxic effects include serious arrhythmias and convulsions, which may be fatal. It is not known how theophylline causes bronchodilatation in asthmatics. Theophylline inhibits phosphodiesterase and increases cellular cAMP levels. The concentration of theophylline that inhibits most phosphodiesterases is higher than the therapeutic range, but there is some evidence that a subtype of the enzyme in airway smooth muscle is more sensitive to the drug.

Cromoglicate

This is a prophylactic drug and is of no value in acute attacks. It has anti-inflammatory actions in some patients but it is not possible to predict which patients will benefit and it is usually less effective than prophylaxis with corticosteroid inhalation. Cromoglicate must be given regularly and it may be several weeks before beneficial effects are apparent. The mechanism of action of cromoglicate is unclear. It may act by decreasing the sensitivity of bronchial sensory nerves, abolishing local reflexes that stimulate inflammation.

Corticosteroids

Steroids effectively increase the airway calibre in asthma by reducing bronchial inflammatory reactions (e.g. oedema and mucus hypersecretion) and by modifying allergic reactions. Oral administration of steroids is associated with many serious adverse effects (Chapter 33) but, except for high doses, these can be avoided in asthma by aerosol administration of the drugs (e.g. **beclometasone**). Inhaled steroids are usually effective in 3–7 days, but oral steroids may be necessary in some patients, where all other therapy fails. Steroid nasal sprays (e.g. **beclometasone**, **budesonide**) are very effective in hay fever and are especially useful in patients with nasal congestion that is not affected by antihistamines.

Acute severe asthma

Oxygen (40–60%) is given together with nebulized or intravenous β_2-agonists (e.g. **salbutamol**). Then intravenous **hydrocortisone** or oral **prednisolone** is given. Nebulized **ipratropium** may also be used if required. If these drugs do not produce a response, an intravenous infusion of aminophylline may help, but there is little evidence that it does. Artificial ventilation may be required.

Antihistamines

Antagonists that block H_1-histamine receptors are used in the treatment of allergic conditions such as hay fever, urticaria, drug sensitivity rashes, pruritus, and insect bites and stings. Older antihistamine drugs (e.g. **chlorphenamine**, **alimemazine**, **promethazine**) have antimuscarinic actions and cross the blood–brain barrier, commonly causing drowsiness and psychomotor impairment. Newer agents (e.g. **loratadine**, **cetirizine**, **fexofenadine**) do not have atropine-like actions and, because they do not cross the blood–brain barrier to any extent, they cause much less drowsiness.

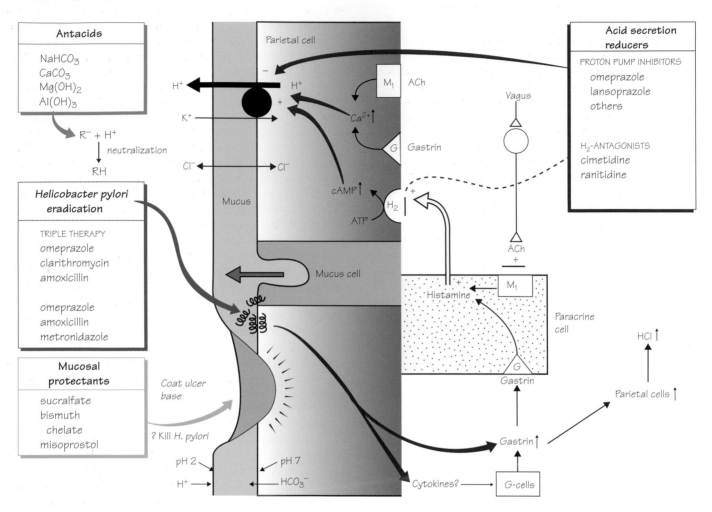

The term **peptic ulcer** refers to any ulcer in an area in which the mucosa is bathed in the hydrochloric acid and pepsin of gastric juice (i.e. the stomach and upper part of the duodenum). Drugs that are effective in the treatment of peptic ulcer either **reduce gastric acid secretion** (left centre and right) or **increase mucosal resistance** to acid–pepsin attack (bottom left).

Acid secretion from the *parietal cells* (⬅) is reduced by **H_2-histamine antagonists** (right) or by **proton pump inhibitors** (right), which can produce virtual anacidity by inhibiting the pump (⬤) that transports H^+ ions out of the parietal cells. Proton pump inhibitors are very effective in promoting ulcer healing, even in patients who are resistant to H_2-antagonists. The '**mucosal protectants**' (bottom left) increase ulcer healing by binding to the ulcer base (left, ▨). This provides **physical protection** and allows the secretion of HCO_3^- to re-establish the pH gradient normally present in the mucus layer (▢) that originates from mucus-secreting cells (⬅). *Misoprostol* is a prostaglandin analogue that promotes ulcer healing by stimulating **protective mechanisms** in the gastric mucosa and by reducing acid

secretion. It is sometimes used to prevent ulcers in patients taking non-steroidal anti-inflammatory drugs (NSAIDs, Chapter 32).

Without continuous drug administration, peptic ulcers, however healed, will often recur. This is because chronic infection of the stomach with *Helicobacter pylori* (〰) is an important aetiological factor in ulcer formation. *H. pylori* infection is associated with about 95% of duodenal ulcers and 70% of gastric ulcers. The infection may result in a chronic hypergastrinaemia, which stimulates acid production and causes ulcers (bottom right). Uncomplicated peptic ulcers associated with *H. pylori* infection are treated by the eradication of *H. pylori* using a combination of a proton pump inhibitor (e.g. omeprazole) with antibiotics (left, centre). Before treatment, infection with *H. pylori* is confirmed by a urea breath test, in which some [13C]urea is ingested. *H. pylori* possesses urease, an enzyme that breaks down the urea and produces [13C]bicarbonate, which can be detected in a sample of breath. The breath test is also used after treatment to verify *H. pylori* eradication.

Antacids (top left) are bases that raise the gastric luminal pH by neutralizing gastric acid (middle left). They provide effective treatment for many dyspepsias and symptomatic relief in peptic ulcer and oesophageal reflux. Many proprietary mixtures, usually containing magnesium or aluminium salts, are available.

Acid secretion

Parietal cells secrete acid into the stomach lumen. This is achieved by a unique H^+/K^+-ATPase (proton pump) that catalyses the exchange of intracellular H^+ for extracellular K^+. The secretion of HCl is stimulated by *acetylcholine* (ACh), released from vagal postganglionic fibres (right of figure), and *gastrin*, released into the bloodstream from G-cells in the antral mucosa when they detect amino acids and peptides (from food) in the stomach, and by gastric distension via local and long reflexes.

Although the parietal cells possess muscarinic (M_1) and gastrin (G) receptors, both ACh and gastrin mainly stimulate acid secretion indirectly by releasing *histamine* from paracrine cells (right, ▨) located close to the parietal cells. Histamine then acts locally (⇐) on the parietal cells, where activation of histamine H_2-receptors (H_2) results in an increase in intracellular cyclic adenosine monophosphate (cAMP) and the secretion of acid. Because ACh and gastrin act indirectly by releasing histamine, the effects on acid secretion of both vagal stimulation and gastrin are reduced by H_2-receptor antagonists.

Cholinergic agonists can powerfully stimulate acid secretion in the presence of H_2-antagonists, indicating that ACh released from the vagus must have limited access to the parietal cell muscarinic receptors. Gastrin acting directly on the parietal cells has a weak effect on acid secretion, but this is greatly potentiated when the histamine receptors are activated.

Protective factors

Mucus layer
This forms a physical barrier (approximately 500 μm thick) on the surface of the stomach and proximal duodenum, and consists of a mucus gel into which HCO_3^- is secreted. Within the gel matrix, the HCO_3^- neutralizes acid diffusing from the lumen. This creates a pH gradient and the gastric mucosa is maintained at a neutral pH, even when the stomach contents are at pH 2. Prostaglandins E_2 and I_2 are synthesized by the gastric mucosa, where they are thought to exert a cytoprotective action by stimulating the secretion of mucus and bicarbonate, and by increasing the mucosal blood flow.

Ulcer healing drugs

Acid secretion reducers

Histamine H_2-receptor antagonists
Cimetidine and **ranitidine** are rapidly absorbed orally. They block the action of histamine on the parietal cells and reduce acid secretion. These drugs relieve the pain of peptic ulcer and increase the rate of ulcer healing. The incidence of side-effects is low. Cimetidine has slight antiandrogenic actions, and rarely causes gynaecomastia. Cimetidine also binds to cytochrome P-450 and may reduce the hepatic metabolism of drugs (e.g. warfarin, phenytoin and theophylline).

Proton pump inhibitors
Omeprazole and **lansoprazole** are inactive at neutral pH, but in acid they rearrange into two types of reactive molecule, which react with

sulphydryl groups in the H^+/K^+-ATPase (proton pump) responsible for transporting H^+ ions out of the parietal cells. Because the enzyme is irreversibly inhibited, acid secretion only resumes after the synthesis of new enzyme. These agents are particularly useful in patients with severe gastric acid hypersecretion caused by Zollinger–Ellison syndrome, a rare condition produced by an islet-cell gastrin-secreting tumour of the pancreas, and in patients with reflux oesophagitis where severe ulceration is usually resistant to other drugs.

H. pylori is a mobile, spiral-shaped, Gram-negative rod found deep in the mucus layer where a pH of 7.0 is optimal for its growth. The bacteria invade the epithelial cell surface to some extent, and toxins and ammonia produced by strong urease activity may damage the cells. Gastritis associated with *H. pylori* infection persists for years, or for life, and is associated with a sustained increase in gastrin release, which increases the basal release of HCl. The increased gastrin release may be caused by cytokines resulting from inflammation, which also compromises mucosal defence. A trophic effect of the hypergastrinaemia increases the mass of the parietal cells causing an exaggerated acid-secreting response to gastrin. In the duodenum, the acid induces mucosal injury and metaplastic cells of the gastric phenotype. Chronic inflammation of these cells leads to ulceration. Eradication of *H. pylori* significantly reduces HCl secretion and produces long-term healing of duodenal and gastric ulcers. Trials have shown that a combination of acid inhibition and antibiotics can eradicate *H. pylori* in over 90% of patients in 1 week. Most recommended drug combinations include clarithromycin, e.g. clarithromycin, omeprazole and metronidazole (or amoxicillin). If clarithromycin cannot be used, amoxicillin, metronidazole and omeprazole may be used. Resistance to metronidazole is common.

Mucosal protectants
Sucralfate polymerizes below pH 4 to give a very sticky gel that adheres strongly to the base of ulcer craters. Bismuth chelate (tripotassium dicitratobismuthate) may act in a similar way to sucralfate. It has a strong affinity for mucosal glycoproteins, especially in the necrotic tissue of the ulcer craters, which become coated in a protective layer of polymer–glycoprotein complex. Bismuth may blacken the teeth and stools. Bismuth and sucralfate must be given on an empty stomach or they will complex with food proteins.

Antacids
Antacids raise the luminal pH of the stomach. This increases the rate of emptying and so the effect of antacids is short-lived. Gastrin release is increased and, because this stimulates acid release, larger amounts of antacids are needed than would be predicted (acid rebound). Frequent high doses of antacids promote ulcer healing, but such treatment is rarely practical.

Sodium bicarbonate is the only useful water-soluble antacid. It acts rapidly but has a transient action, and absorbed bicarbonate in high doses may cause systemic alkalosis.

Magnesium hydroxide and magnesium trisilicate are insoluble in water and have a fairly rapid action. Magnesium has a laxative effect and may cause diarrhoea.

Aluminium hydroxide has a relatively slower action. Al^{3+} ions form complexes with certain drugs (e.g. tetracyclines) and tend to cause constipation. Mixtures of magnesium and aluminium compounds may be used to minimize the effects on motility.

13 Drugs acting on the gastrointestinal tract II: motility and secretions

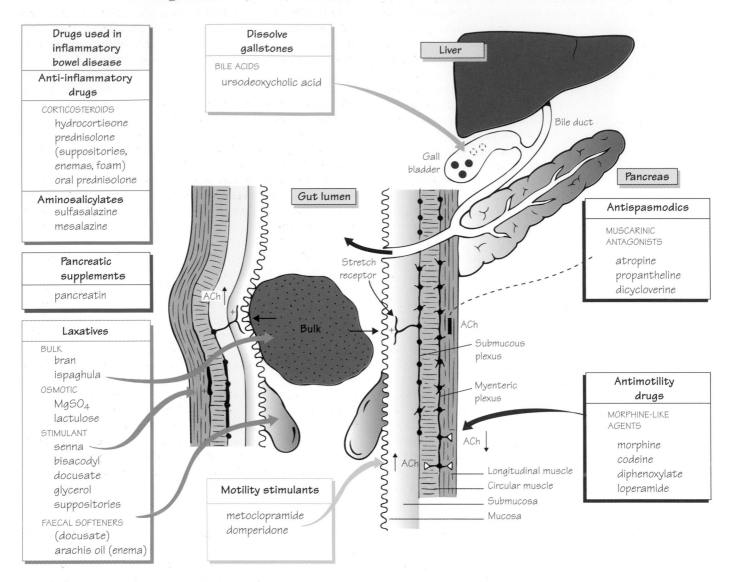

Muscular contractions of the gut and secretion of acid and enzymes are under autonomic control. The enteric part of the autonomic nervous system consists of ganglionated plexuses (⊶) with complex interconnections supplying the smooth muscle, mucosa and blood vessels. The ganglia (⊶) (parasympathetic) receive extrinsic excitatory fibres from the vagus and inhibitory sympathetic fibres. Other transmitters in the gut include 5-hydroxytryptamine (5HT), adenosine triphosphate (ATP), nitric oxide and neuropeptide Y.

Cholinomimetic drugs (e.g. **carbachol**, **neostigmine**) increase motility and may cause colic and diarrhoea. They are very occasionally used in the treatment of paralytic ileus (Chapter 8). More useful **motility stimulants** (bottom middle) facilitate acetylcholine release from the myenteric plexus and are used in the treatment of oesophageal reflux and gastric stasis. **Laxatives** (bottom left) are drugs used to increase the motility of the gut and encourage defecation. **Bulk laxatives** (▨) stimulate stretch receptors in the mucosa. **Stimulant laxatives** stimulate

the myenteric plexus, and some drugs act as **lubricants** (▨). Muscarinic antagonists (top right) reduce gastrointestinal motility and are used to reduce spasm in irritable bowel syndrome (**antispasmodics**). Antidiarrhoeal drugs include **antimotility drugs** (bottom right), but *replacement of water and electrolyte loss is generally more important than drug treatment*, especially in infants and in infectious diarrhoea.

Anti-inflammatory corticosteroids and aminosalicylates (top left) are used in ulcerative colitis and Crohn's disease. To reduce the need for systemic steroids, it is usual to add **azathioprine**, an immunosuppressant (Chapter 44).

In the duodenum, bile from the liver (top right) and pancreatic juice from the pancreas (right, ▨) enter (⬅) usually through a common opening that is restricted by the sphincter of Oddi. **Bile acids** (top middle) are sometimes used to dissolve cholesterol gallstones (●). **Pancreatic supplements** (left middle) are given orally when the secretion of pancreatic juice is absent or reduced.

Motility stimulants

Metoclopramide and **domperidone** are dopamine antagonists and, by blocking central dopamine receptors in the chemoreceptor trigger zone, they produce an antinausea/antiemetic action (see also Chapter 30). The drugs also increase contractions in the stomach and enhance the tone of the lower oesophageal sphincter, actions that combine to speed the transit of contents from the stomach. The prokinetic actions of metoclopramide and domperidone are blocked by atropine, suggesting that they result from an increase of acetylcholine release from the myenteric plexus. This effect on acetylcholine release is thought to be caused by the activation of $5HT_4$ receptors on the cholinergic neurones. **Tegaserod**, a $5HT_4$ partial agonist, causes a modest improvement in some patients with irritable bowel syndrome with predominant constipation. In women with severe irritable bowel syndrome with predominant diarrhoea, the $5HT_3$ antagonist, **alosetron**, may be beneficial. It acts by blocking $5HT_3$ receptors on enteric afferents, blocking reflex contraction of the intestine. Unfortunately, unlike tegaserod, which is very safe, alosetron may cause fatal ischaemic colitis.

Laxatives

Constipation is characterized by abdominal discomfort, loss of appetite and malaise resulting from insufficient frequency of defecation; this results in abnormally hard and dry faeces. The frequency and volume of defecation are best regulated by diet, but drugs may be needed for specific purposes (e.g. before surgery of the colon or rectum; colonoscopy).

Bulk laxatives increase the volume of the intestinal contents, stimulating peristalsis. They include indigestible polysaccharides such as cellulose (bran) and ispaghula. **Osmotic laxatives** increase bulk in the bowel by retaining water by an osmotic effect. They include salts containing poorly absorbed ions (e.g. $MgSO_4$, Epsom salts) and **lactulose**, which takes 48 h to act and must be given regularly.

Stimulant laxatives increase motility by acting on the mucosa or nerve plexuses, which may be damaged by prolonged drug use. They often cause abdominal cramp. Anthraquinones released from precursor glycosides present in **senna** stimulate the myenteric plexus. **Glycerol** suppositories stimulate the rectum because glycerol is mildly irritant. **Bisacodyl** and **sodium picosulfate** may act by stimulating sensory nerve endings. They are mainly used to evacuate the bowel before surgery or endoscopic procedures on the colon.

Faecal softeners promote defecation by softening (e.g. **docusate**) and/or lubricating (e.g. **arachis oil**, **liquid paraffin**) faeces and assisting evacuation. Chronic use of liquid paraffin may impair absorption of the fat-soluble vitamins A and D and cause paraffinomas.

Antidiarrhoeal drugs

Infectious diarrhoea is a very common cause of illness and results in a high mortality in developing countries. Bacterial pathogens cause the most severe forms of infectious diarrhoea, but more often diarrhoea is caused by a viral infection.

Antimotility drugs are widely used to provide symptomatic relief in mild to moderate forms of acute diarrhoea. Opioids such as *morphine*, *diphenoxylate* and *codeine* activate μ-receptors on myenteric neurones and cause hyperpolarization by increasing their potassium conductance. This inhibits acetylcholine release from the myenteric plexus and reduces bowel motility. **Loperamide** is the most appropriate opioid for local effects on the gut because it does not easily penetrate to the brain. Hence, it has few central actions and is unlikely to cause dependence.

Rehydration therapy. Oral solutions containing electrolytes and glucose are given to correct the severe dehydration that can be caused by infection with toxigenic organisms.

Antibiotics are useful only in certain specific infections, e.g. cholera and severe bacillary dysentery, which are treated with tetracycline. The quinolones (Chapter 37) are more recent agents that seem to be effective against most important diarrhoeal pathogens.

Drugs used in inflammatory bowel disease

Inflammatory bowel disease is divided into two types:
1 **Crohn's disease**, which can affect the entire gut; and
2 **ulcerative colitis**, which affects only the large bowel.

Local or systemic anti-inflammatory **corticosteroids**, e.g. **prednisolone** (Chapter 33), are the main drugs used for acute attacks, but their serious adverse effects make them unsuitable for maintenance treatment. However, oral **budesonide** (slow release) is a corticosteroid with reduced absorption and may not cause adrenal suppression. **Aminosalicylates** reduce the symptoms in mild disease, and maintenance treatment reduces the relapse rates of patients in remission. **Sulfasalazine** is a combination of 5-aminosalicylic acid with a sulphonamide that carries the drug to the colon where it is cleaved by bacteria, releasing **5-aminosalicylic acid**, which is the active moiety, and sulfapyridine, which is absorbed and may produce the adverse effects characteristic of sulphonamides (e.g. nausea, rashes, blood disorders; see Chapter 37). Newer, less toxic drugs are **mesalazine**, which is 5-aminosalicylate in a preparation that releases the drug in the colon, and **olsalazine** (azodisalicylate), which consists of two molecules of 5-aminosalicylic acid joined by an azo bond, cleaved by bacteria in the colon. The mechanism of action of 5-aminosalicylate is unknown. Patients who do not respond to steroids or aminosalicylates may benefit from immunosuppressants, e.g. **azathioprine**, **mercaptopurine**, and **methotrexate** (Chapter 44). **Infliximab** is a monoclonal antibody to tumour necrosis factor-α (TNF-α). Inhibition of this proinflammatory cytokine can be very effective in treating severe refractory Crohn's disease.

Drugs used to dissolve gallstones

Bile contains cholesterol and bile salts, the latter being important in keeping cholesterol in solution. An increase in cholesterol concentration or a decrease in bile salts may result in the formation of cholesterol stones. If they give rise to symptoms, laparoscopic cholecystectomy is the treatment of choice. However, small non-calcified stones may be dissolved by prolonged oral administration of the bile acid **ursodeoxycholic acid**, which decreases the cholesterol content of bile by inhibiting an enzyme involved in cholesterol formation.

Pancreatic supplements

Pancreatic juice contains important enzymes that break down proteins (trypsin, chymotrypsin), starch (amylase) and fats (lipase). In some diseases (e.g. chronic pancreatitis, cystic fibrosis), there is an absence or reduction in these enzymes. Patients with pancreatic insufficiency are given **pancreatin**, an extract of pancreas containing protease, lipase and amylase. Because the enzymes are inactivated by gastric acid, it is usual to give an H_2-receptor antagonist (e.g. *cimetidine*) beforehand. Newer enteric-coated preparations that deliver more of the enzymes to the duodenum are available.

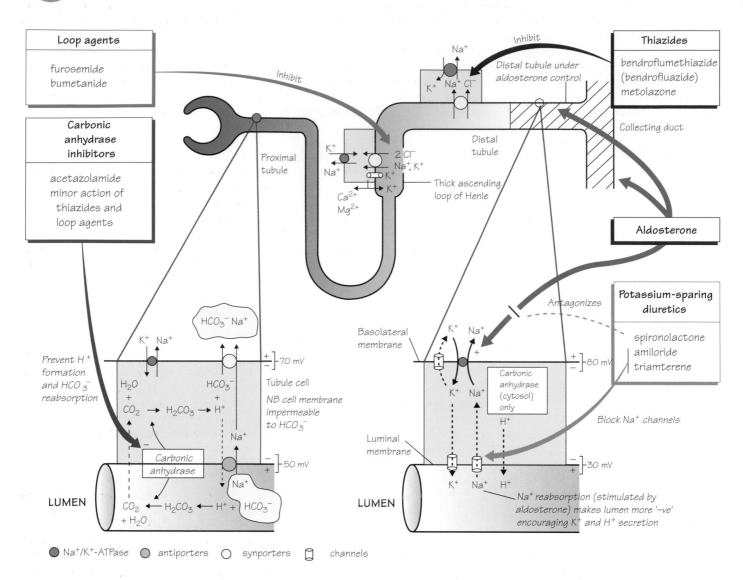

Diuretics are drugs that act on the kidney to increase the excretion of water and sodium chloride. Normally, reabsorption of salt and water is controlled by **aldosterone** and **vasopressin** (antidiuretic hormone, ADH), respectively. Most diuretics work by reducing the reabsorption of electrolytes by the tubules (top). The increased electrolyte excretion is accompanied by an increase in water excretion, necessary to maintain an osmotic balance. Diuretics are used to reduce oedema in *congestive heart failure*, some *renal diseases* and *hepatic cirrhosis*. Some diuretics, notably the thiazides, are widely used in the treatment of hypertension, but their long-term hypotensive action is not only related to their diuretic properties.

The **thiazides** and related compounds (top right) are safe, orally active, but relatively weak diuretics. More effective drugs are the **high ceiling** or **loop diuretics** (top left). These drugs have a very rapid onset and fairly short duration of action. They are very powerful (hence the term 'high ceiling') and can cause serious electrolyte imbalances and dehydration. **Metolazone** is a thiazide-related drug with

activity between the loop and thiazide diuretics. It has a powerful synergistic action with furosemide, and the combination may be effective in resistant oedema and in patients with seriously impaired renal function. The thiazides and the loop diuretics increase potassium excretion, and potassium supplements may be required to prevent hypokalaemia.

Some diuretics are '**potassium sparing**' (bottom right). They are weak when used alone, but they cause potassium retention, and are often given with thiazides or loop diuretics to prevent hypokalaemia.

Carbonic anhydrase inhibitors (bottom left) are weak diuretics and are rarely used for their diuretic action. **Osmotic diuretics** (e.g. *mannitol*) are compounds that are filtered but not reabsorbed. They are excreted with an osmotic equivalent of water and are used in cerebral oedema, and sometimes to maintain a diuresis during surgery.

The kidney is one of the major routes of drug elimination, and impairment of renal function in old age or in renal disease can significantly decrease the elimination of drugs.

Aldosterone stimulates Na^+ reabsorption in the distal tubule and increases K^+ and H^+ secretion. It acts on cytoplasmic receptors (Chapter 33) and induces the synthesis of Na^+/K^+-ATPase in the basolateral membrane and Na^+ channels in the luminal membrane. A more rapid increase in Na^+ channel permeability may be mediated by cell surface aldosterone receptors. Diuretics *increase* the Na^+ load in the distal tubule and, except for the potassium-sparing agents, this results in an *increased K^+ secretion* (and excretion). This effect is greater if plasma aldosterone levels are high; for example, if vigorous diuretic therapy has depleted the body of Na^+ stores.

Vasopressin (**ADH**) is released from the posterior pituitary gland. It increases the number of water channels in the collecting ducts allowing the passive reabsorption of water. In 'cranial' diabetes insipidus, absence of ADH causes the excretion of large volumes of hypotonic urine. This is treated with vasopressin or **desmopressin**, a longer-acting analogue.

Carbonic anhydrase inhibitors depress bicarbonate reabsorption in the proximal tubule by inhibiting the catalysis of CO_2 hydration and dehydration reactions. Thus, the excretion of HCO_3^-, Na^+ and H_2O is increased. The loss of HCO_3^- causes a metabolic acidosis and the effects of the drug become self-limiting as the blood bicarbonate falls. The increased Na^+ delivered to the distal nephron increases K^+ secretion. **Acetazolamide** is used in the treatment of glaucoma to reduce intraocular pressure, which it does by reducing the secretion of HCO_3^- and associated H_2O into the aqueous humour (Chapter 10). It is also used as a prophylactic agent for mountain (altitude) sickness.

Thiazides

Thiazides were developed from the carbonic anhydrase inhibitors. However, the diuretic activity of these drugs is not related to their effects on this enzyme. The thiazides are widely used in the treatment of mild heart failure (Chapter 18) and hypertension (Chapter 15), in which condition they have been shown to reduce the incidence of stroke. There are many thiazides, but the only major difference is their duration of action. **Bendroflumethiazide** is widely used.

Mechanism of action

Thiazides act mainly on the early segments of the *distal tubule*, where they *inhibit NaCl reabsorption* by binding to the synporter responsible for the electroneutral cotransport of Na^+/Cl^-. Excretion of Cl^-, Na^+ and accompanying H_2O is increased. The increased Na^+ load in the distal tubule stimulates Na^+ exchange with K^+ and H^+, increasing their excretion and causing hypokalaemia and a metabolic alkalosis.

Adverse effects

Adverse effects include *weakness*, *impotence* and occasionally *skin rashes*. Serious allergic reactions (e.g. thrombocytopenia) are rare. More common are the following metabolic effects:

1 Hypokalaemia may precipitate cardiac arrhythmias, especially in patients on digitalis. This can be prevented by giving potassium supplements if necessary, or by combined therapy with a potassium-sparing diuretic.

2 Hyperuricaemia. Uric acid levels in the blood are often increased because thiazides are secreted by the organic acid secretory system in the tubules and compete for uric acid secretion. This may precipitate *gout*.

3 Glucose tolerance may be impaired, and thiazides are contraindicated in patients with non-insulin-dependent diabetes.

4 Lipids. Thiazides increase plasma cholesterol levels at least during the first 6 months of administration, but this is of uncertain significance.

Loop diuretics

Loop diuretics (usually **furosemide**) are used orally to reduce peripheral and pulmonary oedema in moderate and severe heart failure (Chapter 18). They are given intravenously to patients with pulmonary oedema that results from acute ventricular failure. Unlike the thiazides, loop diuretics are effective in patients with diminished renal function.

Mechanism of action

Loop agents *inhibit NaCl reabsorption* in the *thick ascending loop of Henle*. This segment has a high capacity for absorbing NaCl and so drugs that act on this site produce a diuresis that is much greater than that of other diuretics. Loop diuretics act on the luminal membrane, where they inhibit the cotransport of $Na^+/K^+/2Cl^-$. (The Na^+ is actively transported out of the cells into the interstitium by an Na^+/K^+-ATPase-dependent pump in the basolateral membrane.) The specificity of the loop diuretics stems from their high local concentration in the renal tubules. However, at high doses, these drugs may induce changes in the electrolyte composition of the endolymph and cause deafness.

Adverse effects

The loop agents may cause hyponatraemia, hypotension, hypovolaemia and hypokalaemia. Potassium loss, as with the thiazides, is often clinically unimportant unless there are additional risk factors for arrhythmias (e.g. digoxin treatment). Calcium and magnesium excretion are increased and hypomagnesaemia may occur. Overenthusiastic use of loop diuretics (high doses, intravenous administration) can cause *deafness*, which may not be reversible.

Potassium-sparing diuretics

These diuretics act on the aldosterone-responsive segments of the distal nephron, where K^+ homeostasis is controlled. *Aldosterone* stimulates Na^+ reabsorption, generating a negative potential in the lumen, which drives K^+ and H^+ ions into the lumen (and hence their excretion). The potassium-sparing diuretics reduce Na^+ reabsorption by either antagonizing aldosterone (**spironolactone**) or blocking Na^+ channels (**amiloride, triamterene**). This causes the electrical potential across the tubular epithelium to fall, reducing the driving force for K^+ secretion. The drugs may cause *severe hyperkalaemia*, especially in patients with renal impairment. Hyperkalaemia is also likely to occur if patients are also taking inhibitors of angiotensin-converting enzyme (e.g. captopril), because these drugs reduce aldosterone secretion (and therefore K^+ excretion).

Spironolactone competitively blocks the binding of aldosterone to its cytoplasmic receptor and so increases the excretion of Na^+ (Cl^- and H_2O) and decreases the 'electrically coupled' K^+ secretion. It is a weak diuretic, because only 2% of the total Na^+ reabsorption is under aldosterone control. Spironolactone is used mainly in liver disease with ascites, Conn's syndrome (primary hyperaldosteronism) and severe heart failure.

Amiloride and **triamterene** decrease the luminal membrane Na^+ permeability in the distal nephron by combining with Na^+ channels and blocking them on a 1:1 basis. This increases Na^+ (Cl^- and H_2O) excretion and decreases K^+ excretion.

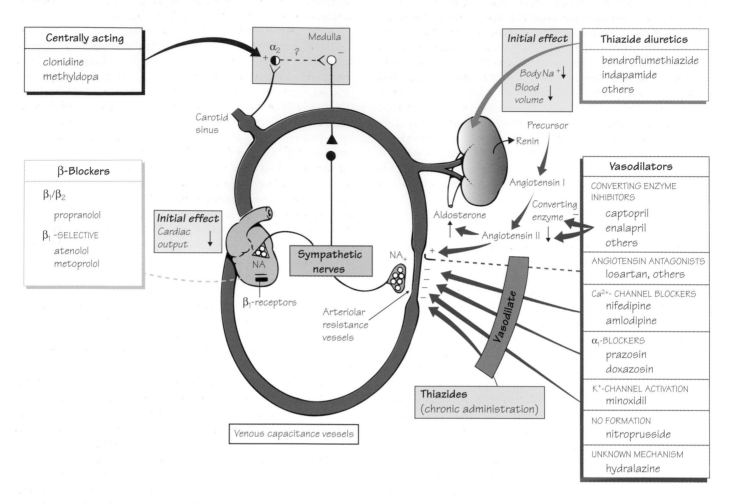

High blood pressure is associated with decreased life expectancy and increased risk of stroke, coronary heart disease and other end-organ disease (e.g. retinopathy, renal failure). The problem is that the risk is graded and so there is no obvious line between patients who should be treated and those who should not. Lowering the blood pressure of patients with a diastolic blood pressure of above 90 mmHg decreases mortality and morbidity, but this could include 25% of the population. In the UK, it is generally accepted that, in patients without additional risk factors, therapy is indicated if the diastolic pressure is greater than 100 mmHg and/or the systolic pressure is greater than 160 mmHg. Other risk factors for vascular disease that may be synergistic include smoking, obesity, hyperlipidaemia, diabetes and left ventricular hypertrophy. A few patients have hypertension secondary to renal or endocrine disease.

In some patients with mild hypertension, increased exercise, weight reduction (if appropriate), reduced alcohol consumption and moderate reduction in salt consumption may be sufficient, but usually drug treatment is required.

Several groups of drugs, by different mechanisms, reduce blood pressure by decreasing vasoconstrictor tone and hence peripheral resistance. The most important of these are the **angiotensin converting enzyme (ACE) inhibitors** (middle right), which decrease circulating angio-tensin II (a vasoconstrictor), **angiotensin II receptor** (AT_1 subtype) **antagonists** and the **calcium-channel blockers** (middle right), which block the entry of calcium into vascular smooth muscle cells. **β-Adrenoceptor antagonists** (β-blockers, centre left) and **thiazide diuretics** (top right) reduce blood pressure by mechanisms that are not fully understood. ACE inhibitors, angiotensin antagonists, calcium-channel blockers and thiazides significantly reduce the risks of stroke, coronary heart disease and cardiovascular death. β-Blockers are equally effective at reducing blood pressure but are less effective than other drugs in reducing the incidence of stroke and myocardial in farction. They are no longer preferred for uncomplicated hypertension but may be used if there are additional indications, e.g. in patients with angina or heart failure, or following myocardial infarction. Other vasodilators (bottom right) have been largely superseded by the ACE inhibitors and calcium antagonists. However, selective α_1 – adrenoceptor antagonists may be used with other drugs in resistant hypertension. **Centrally acting drugs** (top left) are little used because of their adverse effects.

Mild to moderate hypertension may be controlled by a single drug, but most patients require combinations of two or even three drugs adequately to control the blood pressure. The effectiveness of antihypertensive therapy is clear but many, if not most, patients do not have their blood pressure adequately controlled.

Thiazide diuretics

The mechanism by which diuretics reduce arterial blood pressure is not known. Initially, the blood pressure falls because of a decrease in blood volume, venous return and cardiac output. Gradually, the cardiac output returns to normal, but the hypotensive effect remains because the peripheral resistance has, in the meantime, decreased. Diuretics have no direct effect on vascular smooth muscle, and the vasodilatation they cause seems to be associated with a small but persistent reduction in body Na^+. One possible mechanism is that a fall in smooth muscle Na^+ causes a secondary reduction in intracellular Ca^{2+} so that the muscle becomes less responsive to endogenous vasoconstrictors. Thiazide diuretics may cause *hypokalaemia*, *diabetes mellitus* and *gout* (see also Chapter 14), but it is now appreciated that they have a flat dose–response curve and the low doses of thiazides currently used to lower blood pressure cause insignificant metabolic effects. Thiazides seem to be particularly effective in older patients (over 55).

β-Adrenoceptor antagonists

β-Blockers initially produce a fall in blood pressure by decreasing the cardiac output. With continued treatment, the cardiac output returns to normal, but the blood pressure remains low because, by an unknown mechanism, the peripheral vascular resistance is 'reset' at a lower level (individual drugs are discussed in Chapter 9). A central mechanism has been suggested, but this seems unlikely as some drugs do not readily cross the blood–brain barrier. Blockade of $β_1$-receptors in renal juxtaglomerular granule cells that secrete renin may be involved, and such a mechanism could explain why β-blockers are less effective in older patients, who may have low renin levels. Disadvantages of β-blockade are the common adverse effects, such as cold hands and fatigue, and the less common, but serious, adverse effects, such as the *provocation of asthma*, *heart failure* or *conductance block*. β-Blockers also tend to raise serum triglyceride and decrease high-density lipoprotein cholesterol levels. All of the β-blockers lower blood pressure, but at least some of the side-effects can be reduced by using cardioselective hydrophilic drugs (i.e. those without liver metabolism or brain penetration), such as atenolol.

Vasodilator drugs

ACE inhibitors

Angiotensin II is a powerful circulating vasoconstrictor, and inhibition of its synthesis in hypertensive patients results in a fall in peripheral resistance and a lowering of blood pressure. ACE inhibitors do not impair cardiovascular reflexes and are devoid of many of the adverse effects of the diuretics and β-blockers. A common unwanted effect of ACE inhibitors is a dry cough, which may be caused by increased bradykinin (ACE also metabolizes bradykinin). Rare, but serious, adverse effects of ACE inhibitors include angioedema, proteinuria and neutropenia. The first dose may cause a very steep fall in blood pressure, e.g. in patients on diuretics (because they are Na^+ depleted). ACE inhibitors may cause renal failure in patients with bilateral renal artery stenosis, because in this condition angiotensin II is apparently required to constrict postglomerular arterioles and maintain adequate glomerular filtration. Inhibition of angiotensin II formation reduces, but does not seriously impair, aldosterone secretion, and excessive K^+ retention only occurs in patients taking potassium supplements or potassium-sparing diuretics (aldosterone increases Na^+ reabsorption and K^+ excretion; Chapter 14).

Angiotensin receptor antagonists (e.g. **losartan**) lower the blood pressure by blocking angiotensin (AT_1) receptors. They have similar properties to the ACE inhibitors, but do not cause cough, perhaps because they do not prevent bradykinin degradation.

Calcium-channel blockers (see also Chapters 16 and 17). The tone of vascular smooth muscle is determined by the cytosolic Ca^{2+} concentration. This is increased by $α_1$-adrenoceptor activation (resulting from sympathetic tone), which triggers Ca^{2+} release from the sarcoplasmic reticulum via the second messenger inositol-1,4,5-trisphosphate (Chapter 1). There are also receptor-operated cation channels that are important because the entry of cations through them depolarizes the cell, opening voltage-dependent (L-type) Ca^{2+} channels and causing additional Ca^{2+} to enter the cell. The calcium channel blockers (e.g. **nifedipine**, **amlodipine**) bind to the L-type channels and, by blocking the entry of Ca^{2+} into the cell, cause relaxation of the arteriolar smooth muscle. This reduces the peripheral resistance and results in a fall in blood pressure. The efficacy of calcium antagonists is similar to that of the thiazides and ACE inhibitors. Their most common side-effects are caused by excessive vasodilatation and include dizziness, hypotension, flushing and ankle oedema.

α₁-Adrenoceptor antagonists

Prazosin and the longer-acting **doxazosin** cause vasodilatation by selectively blocking vascular $α_1$-adrenoceptors. Unlike non-selective α-blockers, these drugs are not likely to cause tachycardia, but they may cause postural hypotension. They are used with other antihypertensives in cases of resistant hypertension.

Hydralazine is used in combination with a β-blocker and diuretic. Side-effects include reflex tachycardia, which may provoke angina, headaches and fluid retention (as a result of secondary hyperaldosteronism). In slow acetylators in particular, hydralazine may induce a *lupus syndrome* resulting in fever, arthralgia, malaise and hepatitis.

Minoxidil is a potent vasodilator that causes severe fluid retention and oedema. However, when given with a β-blocker and loop diuretic, it is effective in severe hypertension resistant to other drug combinations. Minoxidil relaxes vascular smooth muscle cells by opening adenosine triphosphate (ATP)-sensitive K^+ channels, causing hyperpolarization and closure of voltage-sensitive Ca^{2+} channels. These K^+ channels are normally kept closed by intracellular ATP, which is apparently antagonized by minoxidil sulphate (see oral antidiabetic drugs, Chapter 36).

Centrally acting drugs

Methyldopa is converted in adrenergic nerve endings to the false transmitter, α-methylnorepinephrine, which stimulates $α_2$-receptors in the medulla and reduces sympathetic outflow. Drowsiness is common, and in 20% of patients methyldopa causes a positive antiglobulin (Coombs) test and, rarely, haemolytic anaemia (Chapter 46). **Clonidine** causes rebound hypertension if the drug is suddenly withdrawn.

Acute severe hypertension

In hypertensive crisis, drugs may be given by intravenous infusion (e.g. **hydralazine** in hypertension associated with eclampsia of pregnancy; **nitroprusside** in malignant hypertension with encephalopathy). However, intravenous drugs are rarely necessary, and the trend is to use oral agents whenever possible (e.g. atenolol, amlodipine). Nitroprusside decomposes in the blood to release nitric oxide (NO), an unstable compound that causes vasodilatation (see Chapter 16 for mechanism).

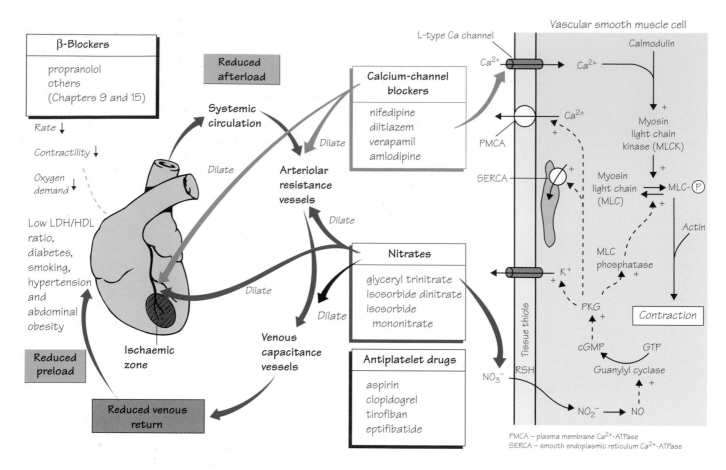

The coronary arteries supply blood to the heart. With increasing age, atheromatous plaques progressively narrow the arteries, and the obstruction to blood flow may eventually become so severe that, when exercise increases the oxygen consumption of the heart, not enough blood can pass through the arteries to supply it. The ischaemic muscle then produces the characteristic symptoms of **angina pectoris** (episodic chest pain that may radiate to the jaw, neck, or arms; shortness of breath; dizziness).

The basic aim of drug treatment of angina is to reduce the work of the heart and hence its oxygen demand. The **nitrates** (middle) are the first-line drugs. Their main effect is to cause peripheral vasodilatation, especially in the veins, by an action on the vascular smooth muscle that involves the formation of nitric oxide (NO) and an increase in intracellular cyclic guanosine monophosphate (cGMP) (right figure). The resulting pooling of blood in the capacitance vessels (veins) reduces venous return, and the end-diastolic ventricular volume is decreased. Reduction in the distension of the heart wall decreases oxygen demand and the pain is quickly relieved. **Glyceryl trinitrate** given sublingually to avoid first-pass metabolism is used to treat acute anginal attacks. If this is required more than twice a week, then combined therapy is required in which **β-adrenoceptor blockers** (top left) or **calcium-channel blockers** (middle top) are taken in addition to glyceryl trinitrate, which is retained for acute attacks.

β-Adrenoceptor blockers depress myocardial contractility and reduce the heart rate. In addition to these effects, which reduce the

oxygen demand, β-blockers may also increase the perfusion of the ischaemic area, because the decrease in heart rate increases the duration of diastole and hence the time available for coronary blood flow. If necessary, a long-acting nitrate is added (middle).

β-Blockers are the standard drugs used in angina, but they have many side-effects and contraindications (Chapter 15). If β-blockers cannot be used, e.g. in patients with asthma, then a **calcium-channel blocker** can be used as an adjunct to short-acting nitrates. Calcium-channel blockers relieve angina mainly by causing peripheral arteriolar dilatation and afterload reduction. They are especially useful if there is some degree of coronary artery spasm (variant angina).

Stable angina occurs when an atheromatous plaque produces a coronary artery stenosis. There is a relatively predictable pattern to the pain, which is usually relieved by rest and nitrates. Patients with stable angina should change their lifestyle (e.g. stop smoking, eat healthily, take more exercise) to try to reduce the progression of atheroma. They should take low-dose aspirin to reduce the probability of platelet aggregation, and statins should be considered to lower low-density lipoprotein cholesterol. **Unstable angina** results from fissuring or erosion of an atheromatous plaque. This causes platelet aggregation and the formation of an intracoronary thrombus, which results in a sudden decrease in blood flow through the artery. Patients with unstable angina are at a high risk of myocardial infarction and are treated as an emergency in hospital. They are given heparin and aspirin to reduce the risk of embolus formation. In patients at high risk of myocardial infarction or in whom medical treatment is not controlling symptoms, revascularization is considered. In high-risk patients with unstable angina, GP11b/111a blockade with eptifibratide or tirofiban (Chapter 19) together with aspirin and heparin reduces short-term mortality, myocardial infarction, and the need for urgent revascularization.

Nitrates

Short-acting nitrates. Glyceryl trinitrate (sublingual tablet or spray) acts for about 30 min. It is more useful in preventing attacks than in stopping them once they have begun. Patches containing glycerol trinitrate (transdermal administration) have a long duration of action (up to 24 h).

Long-acting nitrates are more stable and may be effective for several hours, depending on the drug and preparation used (sublingual, oral, oral sustained-release). **Isosorbide dinitrate** is widely used, but it is rapidly metabolized by the liver. The use of **isosorbide mononitrate**, which is the main active metabolite of the dinitrate, avoids the variable absorption and unpredictable first-pass metabolism of the dinitrate.

Adverse effects. The arterial dilatation produced by the nitrates causes headaches, which frequently limit the dose. More serious side-effects are hypotension and fainting. Reflex tachycardia often occurs, but this is prevented by combined therapy with β-blockers. Prolonged high dosage may cause methaemoglobinaemia as a result of oxidation of haemoglobin.

Mechanism of action. Initial metabolism of these drugs releases nitrite ions (NO_2^-), a process that requires tissue thiols. Within the cell, NO_2^- is converted to nitric oxide (NO), which then activates guanylyl cyclase, causing an increase in the intracellular concentration of cGMP in the vascular smooth muscle cells. cGMP activates protein kinase G (PKG), an enzyme that causes the vascular smooth muscle to relax by several mechanisms. These include: (i) activation of Ca pumps that sequester Ca^{2+} into the smooth endoplasmic reticulum (SERCA) and extrude Ca^{2+} into the extracellular space (PMCA); and (ii) activation of K-channels, causing membrane hyperpolarization that inhibits Ca influx by switching off voltage-dependent Ca-channels. The fall in $[Ca^{2+}]_i$ decreases MCLK activity, and relaxation occurs as light-chain phosphorylation is reduced by MCL-phosphatase, the activity of which is increased by PKG.

Tolerance to nitrates may occur. For example, chronic pentaery-thritol tetranitrate has been shown to produce tolerance to sublingual glyceryl trinitrate, and moderate doses of oral isosorbide dinitrate four times a day produce tolerance with loss of the antianginal effect. However, twice daily dosing of isosorbide dinitrate at 08.00 and 13.00 does not produce tolerance, presumably because the overnight rest allows tissue sensitivity to return by the next day. Tolerance to nitrates is poorly understood, but depletion of sulphydryl group donors may be involved, because tolerance to nitrates *in vitro* can sometimes be reversed by *N*-acetylcysteine. Another possibility is that peroxynitrite formed from NO inhibits cGMP formation from guanosine triphosphate (GTP).

β-Adrenoceptor antagonists

β-Blockers are used for the prophylaxis of angina. The choice of drug may be important. *Intrinsic activity might be a disadvantage* in angina, and the cardioselective β-blockers such as **atenolol** and **metoprolol** are probably the drugs of choice. All β-blockers must be avoided in asthmatics as they may precipitate bronchospasm. The **adverse effects** and contraindications of β-blockers should be reviewed (Chapters 9 and 15).

Calcium-channel blockers

These drugs are widely used in the treatment of angina and have fewer serious side-effects than β-blockers. Calcium-channel blockers inhibit L-type voltage-sensitive calcium channels in arterial smooth muscle, causing relaxation and vasodilatation (Chapter 15). Preload is not significantly affected. Calcium channels in the myocardium and conducting tissues of the heart are also affected by calcium-channel blockers, which produce a negative inotropic effect by reducing calcium influx during the plateau phase of the action potential. However, the dihydropyridines (e.g. **nifedipine**, **amlodipine**) have relatively little effect on the heart because they have a much higher affinity for channels in the inactivated state. Such channels are more frequent in vascular muscle because it is relatively more depolarized than cardiac muscle (membrane potential 50 mV cf. 80 mV). Furthermore, at clinical doses, vasodilatation results in a reflex increase in sympathetic tone that causes a mild tachycardia and counteracts the mild negative inotropic effect. **Amlodipine**, which has a long duration of action, produces less tachycardia than nifedipine. **Verapamil** and, to a lesser extent, **diltiazem** depress the sinus node, causing a mild resting bradycardia. Verapamil binds preferentially to open channels and is less affected by the membrane potential. Conduction in the atrioventricular node is slowed and, because the effect of verapamil (unlike nifedipine) is frequency dependent, it effectively slows the ventricular rate in atrial arrhythmias (Chapter 17). The negative inotropic effects of verapamil and diltiazem are partially offset by the reflex increase in adrenergic tone and the decrease in afterload. Diltiazem has actions intermediate between those of verapamil and nifedipine and is popular in the treatment of angina because it does not cause tachycardia.

Tobacco smoking. Smoking is prothrombotic and atherogenic; it reduces coronary blood flow, and the nicotine-induced rise in heart rate and blood pressure increases the oxygen demand of the heart. In addition, the formation of carboxyhaemoglobin reduces the oxygen-carrying capacity of the blood. Some patients improve remarkably on giving up smoking.

Revascularization

Coronary artery bypass grafting (**CABG**) or **percutaneous coronary intervention** (**PCI**) may be indicated in patients not responding to drugs. Generally in bypass operations, the distal end of the internal mammary artery is inserted at a point beyond the stenosis of the affected coronary artery. Angina is relieved or improved in 90% of patients, but returns within 7 years in 50%. Mortality is decreased in some pathological conditions (e.g. left main coronary artery disease). Originally, in PCI, a balloon catheter was used to split and compress the atheromatous plaque, but now the dilatation is followed by a metal wire-mesh tube (stent) to scaffold the vessel segment. Unfortunately, this damages the vessel, often leading to proliferative growth of smooth muscle and restenosis in 20–30% of patients. This problem is significantly reduced by the use of stents that elute sirolimus or paclitaxel from a polymer–drug matrix bound to the stent (less than 10% restenosis rate). Prolonged and continuous antiplatelet therapy is essential with drug-eluting stents because the endothelialization of the stent (which prevents thrombosis) is delayed by the antiproliferative drugs. Unfortunately the ideal duration of antiplatelet therapy (aspirin with clopideral) with drug eluting stents is unkown but is probably at least 12 months.

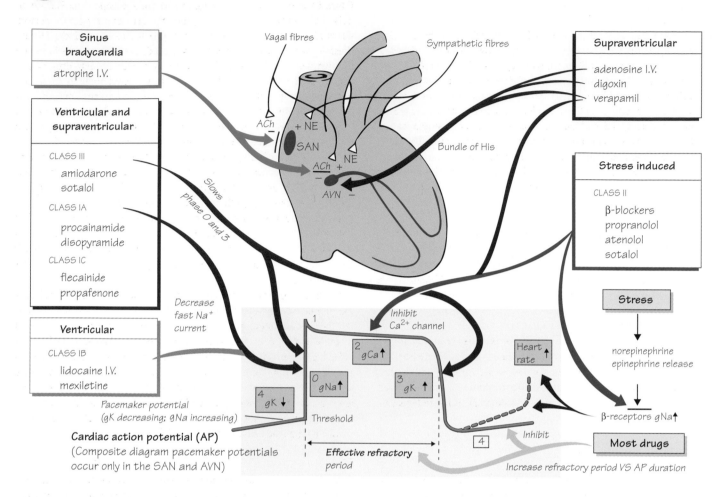

Sinus bradycardia

atropine I.V.

Ventricular and supraventricular

CLASS III
amiodarone
sotalol

CLASS IA
procainamide
disopyramide

CLASS IC
flecainide
propafenone

Ventricular

CLASS IB
lidocaine I.V.
mexiletine

Supraventricular

adenosine I.V.
digoxin
verapamil

Stress induced

CLASS II
β-blockers
propranolol
atenolol
sotalol

Stress

norepinephrine
epinephrine release

β-receptors gNa↑

Most drugs

Vagal fibres

Sympathetic fibres

ACh − + NE

SAN

Bundle of His

ACh − + NE

AVN −

Slows Phase 0 and 3

Decrease fast Na⁺ current

Inhibit Ca²⁺ channel

1

2 gCa↑

0 gNa↑

3 gK↑

4 gK↓

Heart rate ↑

Threshold

Pacemaker potential
(gK decreasing; gNa increasing)

4

Inhibit

Increase refractory period VS AP duration

Cardiac action potential (AP)
(Composite diagram pacemaker potentials
occur only in the SAN and AVN)

Effective refractory period

The rhythm of the heart is normally determined by **pacemaker** cells in the sinoatrial node (SAN, top), but it can be disturbed in a variety of ways, producing anything from occasional discomfort to the symptoms of heart failure or even sudden death. Arrhythmias can occur in the apparently healthy heart, but serious ones (e.g. ventricular tachycardia) are usually associated with heart disease (e.g. myocardial infarction) and a poor prognosis. The rhythm of the heart is affected by both **acetylcholine** (ACh) and **norepinephrine** (NE, noradrenaline), released from parasympathetic and sympathetic nerves, respectively (upper figure).

Supraventricular arrhythmias arise in the atrial myocardium or atrioventricular node (AVN), whereas ventricular arrhythmias originate in the ventricles. Arrhythmias may be caused by an **ectopic focus**, which starts firing at a higher rate than the normal pacemaker (SAN). More commonly, a **re-entry** mechanism is involved, where action potentials, delayed for some pathological reason, re-invade nearby muscle fibres which, being no longer refractory, again depolarize, establishing a loop of depolarization (circus movement).

Many antiarrhythmic drugs have local anaesthetic activity (i.e. block voltage-dependent Na⁺ channels) or are calcium channel blockers. These actions decrease the automaticity of pacemaker cells and increase the effective refractory period of atrial, ventricular and Purkinje fibres.

Antiarrhythmic agents can be classified into:
1 those effective in **supraventricular arrhythmias** (top right);
2 those effective in **ventricular arrhythmias** (bottom left); and

3 those effective in **both types** (middle left).

Arrhythmias associated with stress conditions in which there is an increase in adrenergic activity (emotion, excitement, thyrotoxicosis, myocardial infarction) may be treated with β-blockers (bottom right). An arrhythmia common after acute myocardial infarction is sinus bradycardia, which can be treated with intravenous atropine if the cardiac output is lowered (top left). Antiarrhythmics have also been classified on the basis of their electrophysiological effects on Purkinje fibres (roman numerals). The effects of antiarrhythmic agents on the **cardiac action potential** are shown in the lower figure, but it is not usually known how these actions relate to the drugs' therapeutic effects. Many antiarrhythmic drugs can actually induce lethal arrhythmias, especially in patients with ischaemic heart disease. Except for β-blockers and perhaps amiodarone in myocardial infarction, there is no evidence that antiarrhythmic drugs reduce mortality in any condition. Because of the limitations and dangers of antiarrhythmic drugs, invasive procedures and devices are increasingly being used in serious arrhythmias as **alternatives to drugs**.

Cardiac action potential

Most cardiac cells have two depolarizing currents, a fast Na⁺ current and a slower Ca²⁺ current. However, in the SAN and AVN, there is only a Ca²⁺ current and, because pure 'Ca²⁺ spikes' conduct very slowly, there is a delay between atrial and ventricular contraction. The long refractory period of cardiac fibres normally protects them from re-excitation during a heart beat.

Pacemaker cells

In the SAN and AVN there are no fast channels, and the upswing (essentially phase 2) of the action potential is slow because the depolarization is produced by Ca^{2+} entering through slowly activating L-type Ca^{2+} channels. The pacemaker potential depends on several currents, including an outward K^+ current, which gradually decreases, and two inward Na^+ currents (I_f and I_b), which are relatively stable. As the K^+ current decreases, the Na^+ currents cause increasing depolarization until threshold is reached and an action potential is initiated. The slope of the pacemaker potentials in the SAN is greater than in the AVN, and so the SAN normally determines the heart rate (sinus rhythm). The pacemaker and conducting cells receive autonomic innervation.

Acetylcholine

Vagal fibres release ACh onto M_2-muscarinic receptors that open a K^+ channel (K_{ACh}) via G-protein coupling. The increase in K^+ conductance causes a hyperpolarizing current and decreases the slope of the pacemaker potential. Thus, the threshold for firing is reached later and the heart beat slows. ACh also inhibits atrioventricular conduction.

Norepinephrine

Sympathetic fibres release norepinephrine onto β_1-receptors in the pacemaker tissues and myocardium. Norepinephrine increases the inward Na^+ current (I_f), and so threshold is reached earlier and the heart rate increases. Norepinephrine also increases the force of contraction by increasing the influx of calcium during the plateau phase (positive inotropic effect).

Drugs used in supraventricular arrhythmias

Adenosine stimulates A_1-adenosine receptors and opens ACh-sensitive K^+ channels. This hyperpolarizes the cell membrane in the AVN and, by inhibiting the calcium channels, slows conduction in the AVN. Adenosine is rapidly inactivated ($t_{1/2} = 8$–10 s) and so side-effects (e.g. dyspnoea, bronchospasm) are short-lived. Intravenous adenosine is used to terminate paroxysmal supraventricular tachycardia.

Digoxin stimulates vagal activity (Chapter 18), causing the release of ACh, which slows conduction and prolongs the refractory period in the AVN and bundle of His. Oral administration of digoxin is used in atrial fibrillation, where the atria beat at such high rates that the ventricles can only follow irregularly. By delaying atrioventricular conductance, digoxin increases the degree of block and slows and strengthens the ventricular beat. Intravenous digoxin is used in the treatment of rapid uncontrolled atrial flutter and fibrillation.

Verapamil acts by blocking L-type calcium channels (**class IV agents**) (see also Chapters 15 and 16) and has particularly powerful effects on the AVN, where conduction is entirely dependent on calcium spikes. It also inhibits the influx of Ca^{2+} during the plateau phase of the action potential and therefore has a negative inotropic action. Adenosine has largely replaced intravenous verapamil for the treatment of supraventricular tachycardias because it is safer, especially if the patient really has a ventricular tachycardia, in which case the negative inotropic effect of verapamil may be disastrous. Oral verapamil is still used in the prophylaxis of supraventricular tachycardia. Verapamil should not be used with β-blockers or quinidine because of cumulative negative inotropic effects.

Drugs effective in supraventricular and ventricular arrhythmias

Class IA agents act by blocking (open) voltage-dependent Na^+ channels. They slow phase 0 and lengthen the effective refractory period. Class IA agents produce a frequency (use)-dependent block. During diastole, when the Na^+ channels are closed, class IA agents dissociate relatively slowly (< 5 s) and so, if the frequency is high, drug is still bound to the channel, which therefore cannot contribute to the action potential. **Disopyramide** is mainly used orally to prevent recurrent ventricular arrhythmias. Disopyramide has a negative inotropic action and may cause hypotension (especially intravenously) and aggravate cardiac failure. Other side-effects include nausea, vomiting and marked anticholinergic effects, which may limit its use in men (urinary retention). **Procainamide** is similar to disopyramide but has less antimuscarinic action. It is given intravenously to treat ventricular arrhythmias, especially after myocardial infarction.

Class IC agents dissociate very slowly from Na^+ channels (10–20 s) and strongly depress conduction in the myocardium. **Flecainide** is mainly used in the prophylaxis of paroxysmal atrial fibrillation, but it has a negative inotropic action and may cause serious ventricular arrhythmias.

Class III agents act by slowing repolarization (phase 3) and prolonging the action potential and refractory period in all cardiac tissues. **Amiodarone** has blocking actions on several channels (e.g. K^+ and inactivated Na^+ channels) and β-adrenoceptors. Amiodarone is often effective when other drugs have failed, but its use is restricted to patients in whom other drugs are ineffective because it may cause serious adverse effects, including photosensitivity, thyroid disorders, neuropathy and pulmonary alveolitis. **Sotalol** has class III actions as well as class II (β-blocking) actions. It lacks the side-effects of amiodarone but has the usual side-effects of β-blockers.

Drugs used in ventricular arrhythmias

Class IB agents block (inactivated) voltage-dependent Na^+ channels. **Lidocaine** given intravenously is used in the treatment of ventricular arrhythmias, usually after an acute myocardial infarction. In contrast to class IA agents, which block open Na^+ channels, lidocaine blocks mainly inactivated Na^+ channels. In normal cardiac tissue, lidocaine has little effect because it dissociates rapidly (< 0.5 s) from the Na^+ channels, which therefore recover during diastole. However, in ischaemic areas, where anoxia causes depolarization and arrhythmogenic activity, many Na^+ channels are inactivated and therefore susceptible to lidocaine.

Alternatives to drugs

Pacemakers are required for complete heart block, and are sometimes used in tachyarrhythmias. When the left atrial size is normal, direct current shock causes reversion to sinus rhythm in most patients with atrial fibrillation, but about 60% relapse within 1 year, despite maintenance treatment with disopyramide. Surgical ablation of the ectopic focus or bundle of His is a successful method of controlling supraventricular arrhythmias. A much safer method is ablation of the focus or bundle via electrodes on an intracardiac catheter (endocavity ablation). Because atrioventricular block is produced, a permanent pacemaker is required. In those patients at risk of life-threatening tachyarrhythmias, an implantable automated cardioverter defibrillator may be inserted.

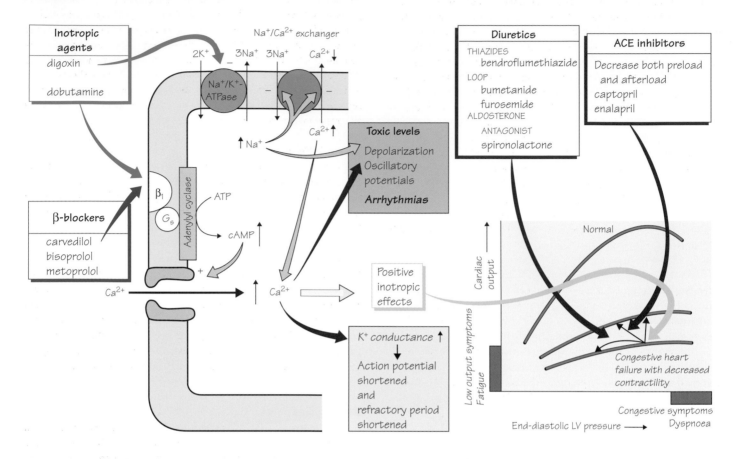

Heart failure exists when the cardiac output is insufficient adequately to perfuse the tissues, despite normal filling of the heart. This leads to a variety of symptoms, e.g. fatigue, oedema, breathlessness and reduced exercise tolerance. *Congestive heart failure* is usually taken to mean combined right and left heart failure, producing both pulmonary congestion and peripheral oedema. Causes of heart failure include hypertension, valvular disease, cardiomyopathy and, most commonly, coronary heart disease. The low cardiac output in heart failure results in increased sympathetic nervous activity, which stimulates the rate and force of the heart beat and maintains the blood pressure by increasing the vascular resistance. In the failing heart, the resulting increase in the resistance against which the heart has to pump (afterload) further depresses cardiac output. Reduced renal blood flow results in *renin secretion* and increased plasma *angiotensin* and *aldosterone* levels. Sodium and water retention increase the blood volume, increasing the central venous pressure (preload) and the likelihood of oedema formation. These compensatory changes at first help to maintain cardiac output but, in the longer term, lead to changes (e.g. abnormal ventricular dilatation) that increase morbidity and mortality. Only drugs that inhibit the neurohormones involved in these compensatory changes increase survival in patients with chronic heart failure (i.e. ACE inhibitors, β-blockers).

Treatment of mild heart failure usually starts with an **angiotensin converting enzyme (ACE) inhibitor** (top right). ACE inhibitors (e.g.

captopril) reduce the load on the heart (diagonal arrow, right figure) and clinical trials have shown that they decrease symptoms, slow disease progression and prolong life in chronic heart failure. In more severe failure, a diuretic (Chapter 14) is added, which increases the excretion of sodium and water and, by reducing the circulating volume, decreases the preload and oedema (curved arrow, right figure). A thiazide (e.g. **bendroflumethiazide**) may be sufficient, but often a loop diuretic is necessary (e.g. **furosemide**). If heart failure is so severe that a combination of diuretic and ACE inhibitor fails to provide an adequate response, then **digoxin**, an **inotropic drug** (top left), may be added. Inotropic drugs all increase the force of cardiac muscle contraction (vertical arrow, right figure) by increasing the rise in cytosolic calcium that occurs with each action potential (left figure). Digoxin increases intracellular calcium indirectly by inhibiting membrane Na^+/K^+-ATPase (⬤). Inotropic drugs all tend to cause arrhythmias because excessive cytosolic calcium can trigger arrhythmogenic membrane currents.

In mild/moderate and severe heart failure, the addition of a **β-blocker** (bottom left) further decreases mortality in patients taking ACE inhibitors and diuretics (with or without digoxin). In patients with severe heart failure and with symptoms uncontrolled with standard therapy, the addition of **spironolactone** (Chapter 14) has been shown to reduce mortality. **Eplerenone** is an alternative aldosterone antagonist that lacks the antiandrogenic effects of spironolactone.

ACE inhibitors

Venous dilatation reduces the filling pressure (preload) and arteriolar dilatation lowers the afterload. The reduction in vascular tone decreases the work and oxygen demand of the failing heart. ACE inhibitors (e.g. **captopril**, **enalapril**) (see also Chapter 15) are the most appropriate vasodilators in heart failure, because they lower both the arterial and venous resistance by preventing the increase in (vasoconstrictor) angiotensin II that is often present in heart failure. The cardiac output increases and, because the renovascular resistance falls, there is an increase in renal blood flow. This latter effect, together with reduced aldosterone release (angiotensin II is a stimulus for aldosterone release), increases Na^+ and H_2O excretion, contracting the blood volume and reducing venous return to the heart. ACE inhibition also reduces the direct growth action that angiotensin has on the heart. Angiotensin antagonists (e.g. **losartan**) may be used as an alternative in patients who cannot tolerate ACE inhibitors, but high doses may be required. Other vasodilators (e.g. isosorbide mononitrate with hydralazine) are now only used in patients who cannot tolerate ACE inhibitors.

β-Blockers

Acutely, β-blockers can decrease myocardial contractility and worsen heart failure. However, long-term administration has been convincingly shown to improve the survival of stable patients with heart failure, presumably by blocking the damaging effects of overactive sympathetic activity. To avoid adverse effects, therapy is started with a low dose that is gradually increased over a period of weeks or months. **Carvedilol**, **bisoprolol** and **metoprolol**, given with an ACE inhibitor and diuretic for about 1 year, have been found in clinical trials to reduce mortality from 11–17% to 7–12%.

Inotropic drugs

Digoxin, a glycoside extracted from leaves of foxglove (*Digitalis* sp.), is the most important inotrope.

Mechanical effects and therapeutic benefit

Digoxin increases the force of cardiac contraction in the failing heart. This benefit has often been doubted in patients with chronic heart failure in sinus rhythm, but recent clinical trials have shown that digoxin can reduce the symptoms of heart failure in patients who are already receiving diuretics and ACE inhibitors. Digoxin is particularly indicated in heart failure caused by atrial fibrillation (Chapter 17).

Mechanism of action

Digoxin inhibits membrane Na^+/K^+-ATPase (⚫), which is responsible for Na^+/K^+ exchange across the muscle cell membrane. This increases intracellular Na^+ and produces a secondary increase in intracellular Ca^{2+} that increases the force of myocardial contraction. The increase in intracellular Ca^{2+} occurs because the decreased Na^+ gradient across the membrane reduces the extrusion of Ca^{2+} by the Na^+/Ca^{2+} exchanger (⚫) that occurs during diastole.

Digoxin and K^+ ions compete for a 'receptor' (Na^+/K^+-ATPase) on the outside of the muscle cell membrane, and so the effects of digoxin may be *dangerously increased in hypokalaemia*, produced, for example, by diuretics.

Electrical effects

These are due to a complicated mixture of direct and indirect actions.

Direct effects (bottom, ☐)

In atrial and ventricular cells, the action potential and refractory period are shortened, because the increased intracellular Ca^{2+} stimulates the potassium channels. Toxic concentrations (top, ◼) cause depolarization (resulting from Na^+ pump inhibition), and oscillatory depolarizing afterpotentials appear after normal action potentials (caused by increased intracellular Ca^{2+}). If these delayed afterpotentials reach threshold, action potentials are generated, causing 'ectopic beats'. With increasing toxicity, the ectopic beat itself elicits further beats, causing a self-sustaining arrhythmia (ventricular tachycardia), which may progress to ventricular fibrillation.

Indirect effects

Digoxin increases central vagal activity and facilitates muscarinic transmission in the heart. This (i) slows the heart rate; (ii) slows atrioventricular conductance; and (iii) prolongs the refractory period of the atrioventricular node. *Use is made of this effect in atrial fibrillation* (Chapter 17), but at toxic levels heart block occurs.

Effects on other organs

Digoxin affects all excitable tissues, its cardioselectivity resulting from a greater dependence of myocardial function on the rate of sodium extrusion. The most common extracardiac action is on the gut, and digoxin may cause anorexia, nausea, vomiting or diarrhoea. These effects are partly brought about by actions on the smooth muscle of the gut and are partly a result of central vagal and chemoreceptor trigger zone stimulation. Less common effects include confusion or even psychosis.

Toxicity

Digoxin toxicity is *quite common* because arrhythmias can occur at concentrations only two or three times that of the optimal therapeutic concentration. According to its severity, treatment may require withdrawal of the drug, potassium supplements, antiarrhythmic drugs (phenytoin or lidocaine) or, in very severe intoxication, digoxin-specific antibody fragments (Fab).

Sympathomimetic agents

These activate cardiac β-receptors and stimulate adenylyl cyclase, an effect mediated by a G-protein called G_s (left). The resulting rise in cyclic adenosine monophosphate (cAMP) activates cAMP-dependent protein kinase, which leads to phosphorylation of the L-type Ca^{2+} channels and an increase in the probability of their opening. This increases the influx of Ca^{2+} and hence the force of myocardial contraction. In contrast to digoxin, which has a neutral effect on survival, other positive inotropes have been found to increase mortality. For this reason, non-glycoside inotropes are used only short term in refractory patients or those awaiting cardiac transplantation. **Dobutamine** is given by intravenous infusion in *acute severe heart failure*. It stimulates $β_1$-adrenoceptors in the heart and increases contractility with little effect on rate. In addition, an action on $β_2$-receptors causes vasodilatation. **Dopamine** given by intravenous infusion in low doses to healthy volunteers increases renal perfusion by stimulating dopamine receptors in the renal vasculature. This finding has long encouraged the use of low doses of dopamine (together with dobutamine) in cardiogenic shock, where deterioration of renal function is common. However, a clinical trial found no benefit in critically ill patients given low-dose dopamine.

19 Drugs used to affect blood coagulation

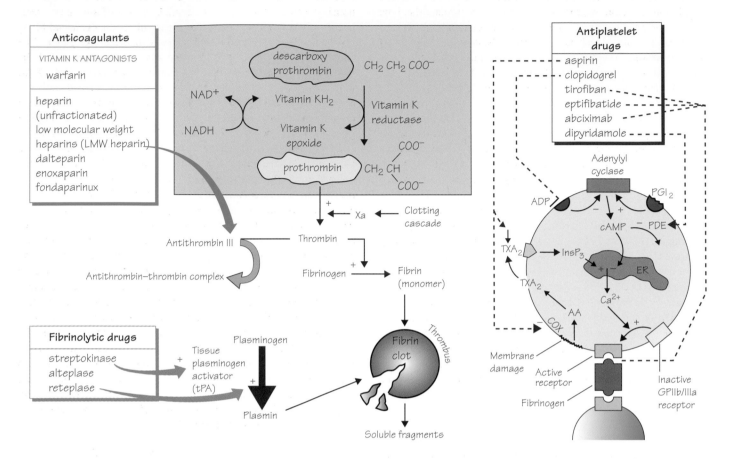

The centre of the figure shows the final stages of the cascade sequence involved in clot (thrombus) formation. In the slower moving venous side of the circulation, the thrombus (⬤) consists of a fibrin web enmeshed with platelets and red blood cells. **Anticoagulant drugs** (top left), particularly heparin and warfarin, are widely used in the prevention and treatment of *venous thrombosis* and *embolism* (e.g. deep vein thrombosis, prevention of postoperative thrombosis, atrial fibrillation, patients with artificial heart valves). The main adverse effect of anti-coagulants is *haemorrhage*.

Heparin is short acting and must be given by injection. Its anti-coagulant effect requires the presence of *antithrombin III*, a pro-tease inhibitor in the blood that forms a 1:1 complex with thrombin (⟹). Heparin increases the *rate* of complex formation 1000-fold, causing the almost instantaneous inactivation of thrombin. The heparin–antithrombin III complex also inhibits factor Xa and some other factors. Low molecular weight (LMW) heparin–antithrombin complex inhibits only factor Xa. Heparin acts both *in vitro* and *in vivo*.

Warfarin is active orally. It is a coumarin derivative with a structure similar to that of vitamin K. Warfarin inhibits vitamin K reductase and blocks vitamin K-dependent γ-carboxylation of glutamate residues (top, shaded), resulting in the production of modified factors VII, IX, X and prothrombin (II). These are inactive in promoting coagulation because the γ-carboxylation confers Ca^{2+}-binding properties that are essential for the proteins to assemble into an efficient catalytic complex. The oral anticoagulants are only active *in vivo* and take 2–3 days for the full anticoagulant effect to develop. Thus, if an immediate effect is required, heparin must be given in addition.

Anticoagulants are less useful in preventing *arterial thrombosis*, because in faster flowing vessels thrombi are composed mainly of platelets with little fibrin. **Antiplatelet drugs** (right) reduce platelet aggregation and arterial thrombosis. In atheromatous arteries, the plaques most likely to rupture possess a large lipid-rich core covered by a thin fibrous cap. Rupture of the cap exposes subendothelial collagen that activates platelets and causes aggregation. This releases thromboxane-A_2 (TXA_2), adenosine diphosphate (ADP) and 5-hydroxytryptamine (5HT) (right figure), which promote further platelet aggregation, vaso-constriction and activation of the clotting cascade. Antiplatelet drugs, especially aspirin, have been shown to reduce the risk of myocardial infarction in patients with unstable angina, increase the survival of patients who have had myocardial infarction and reduce the risk of stroke in patients with transient ischaemic attacks.

Fibrinolytic drugs (bottom left) are administered intravenously. They are agents that can rapidly lyse thrombi by activating plasmino-gen to form plasmin (⬇), which is a proteolytic enzyme that degrades fibrin and so dissolves thrombi. Thrombolytic drugs, especially strep-tokinase, are extensively used together with oral aspirin in the treatment of myocardial infarction, and all have been shown to decrease mortality. The beneficial effects are greatest if the drugs are given within 30 min of myocardial infarction, with progressively less benefit over 24 h. Rapid administration of a thrombolytic agent after infarction is more important than the choice of agent.

Thrombus is an unwanted clot inside a blood vessel. Thrombosis is particularly likely to occur where the blood flow is sluggish, because this allows activated clotting factors to accumulate instead of being washed away. A common problem is postoperative thrombosis in the leg veins. Sometimes bits of thrombus break off (emboli) and are carried to distant sites, which may be severely damaged, e.g. pulmonary embolism. In atrial fibrillation, the loss of atrial contraction predisposes to stasis of blood and encourages thrombus formation. These thrombi may detach and cause cerebral embolism (stroke).

Anticoagulants

Heparin is a naturally occurring, highly acidic glycosaminoglycan of varying molecular weight (5000–15 000). Subcutaneous injections or continuous intravenous infusions of heparin reduce the incidence of deep venous thrombosis in patients undergoing general surgery and those recovering from stroke and myocardial infarction.

The main side-effect of heparin is bleeding. Because it has a short duration of action (4–6 h), bleeding can usually be controlled by stopping drug administration. If necessary, heparin can be neutralized by the intravenous injection of protamine, a basic peptide that combines with the acidic heparin. Heparin occasionally causes allergic reactions and thrombocytopenia.

Low molecular weight heparins have a longer half-life than standard heparin. They have largely replaced unfractionated heparin because they require only a single daily dose by subcutaneous injection, prophylactic doses do not require monitoring, and thrombocytopenia is rare.

Fondaparinux is a synthetic pentasaccharide that binds to antithrombin with high specificity and inhibits factor Xa. It may be superior to LMW heparins.

Vitamin K antagonists

Warfarin is well absorbed after oral administration, but the onset of its full anticoagulant effect is delayed for 2–3 days, while the inactive coagulation factors induced by the drug gradually replace those originally present. Warfarin has a long half-life (about 40 h) and it can take up to 5 days for the prothrombin time to return to normal after stopping treatment. It is metabolized by the liver to inactive 7-hydroxywarfarin. Drugs that induce hepatic microsomal enzymes (e.g. *barbiturates*, *carbamazepine*) antagonize the anticoagulant action of warfarin, and haemorrhage may occur if they are withdrawn. Drugs that inhibit hepatic enzymes decrease the catabolism of warfarin and potentiate its action (e.g. *cimetidine*, *ethanol*, *metronidazole*). Warfarin can be reversed by giving a concentrate of clotting factors (or fresh frozen plasma, which contains clotting factors); this is the treatment of choice for rapid reversal. In severe overdosage, vitamin K (phytomenadione) can be given by intravenous injection, but it takes 6–12 h to act.

Antiplatelet drugs

The key event in platelet activation and aggregation is an increase in cytoplasmic calcium. This causes a conformational change of the inactive glycoprotein GPIIb/IIIa receptors (☐) on the plasma membrane to receptors with a high affinity for fibrinogen (▮), which forms cross-links between the platelets, and hence aggregation. TXA$_2$, thrombin and 5HT activate phospholipase C, and the resulting inositol-1,4,5-trisphosphate (InsP$_3$) stimulates calcium release from the endoplasmic reticulum (ER). ADP inhibits adenylyl cyclase and the decrease in cyclic adenosine monophosphate (cAMP) again increases cytoplasmic calcium. All antiplatelet drugs act one way or another to inhibit these calcium-dependent pathways of platelet activation.

Aspirin reduces the risk of myocardial infarction in patients with unstable angina and increases survival in patients who have had acute myocardial infarction. It also reduces the risk of stroke in patients with transient ischaemic attacks. The beneficial effects of aspirin in thromboembolic disease are brought about by the inhibition of platelet TXA$_2$ synthesis. TXA$_2$ is a powerful inducer of platelet aggregation. The endothelial cells of the vascular wall produce a prostaglandin, PGI$_2$ (prostacyclin), which may be the physiological antagonist of TXA$_2$. PGI$_2$ stimulates different receptors on the platelet and activates adenylyl cyclase. The resulting increase in cAMP causes a decrease in cytoplasmic calcium and inhibition of platelet aggregation. Aspirin prevents TXA$_2$ formation by irreversibly inhibiting cyclooxygenase (COX) (Chapter 32). Platelets cannot synthesize new enzyme, but the vascular endothelial cells can, and a low dose (75–300 mg) of aspirin given daily produces a selective inhibition of cyclo-oxygenase over much of the dose interval. Thus, the balance of the anti-aggregatory effects of PGI$_2$ and the pro-aggregatory effects of TXA$_2$ is shifted in a beneficial direction. **Clopidogrel**, a thienopyridine derivative, reduces aggregation by irreversibly blocking the effects of ADP on platelets. It has a synergistic action when given with aspirin, the latter drug having a relatively weak antiplatelet action on its own. Clopidogrel is also used in patients for whom aspirin is contraindicated. **Eptifibatide**, **tirofiban** and **abciximab** (a monoclonal antibody) inhibit platelet aggregation by binding to the GPIIb/IIIa receptors. They are given by intravenous infusion, together with aspirin and heparin, to prevent myocardial infarction in high-risk patients with unstable angina awaiting percutaneous coronary intervention (PCI). **Dipyridamole** is used with warfarin to prevent thrombosis formation on prosthetic heart valves, although there is doubt about its efficacy. It is thought to reduce platelet aggregation by increasing cAMP levels. (It is a phosphodiesterase inhibitor, but may stimulate adenylyl cyclase.)

Fibrinolytic drugs (thrombolytics)

Fibrinolytic drugs are used extensively in cases of myocardial infarction to lyse the thrombi that block coronary arteries. They are administered by intravenous infusion and probably cause reperfusion in about 50% of arteries if given within 3 h. *The beneficial effects of aspirin in myocardial infarction are additive to those of thrombolytics.* The main side-effects of thrombolytics are bleeding, nausea, vomiting and, in the case of streptokinase, allergic reactions. Bleeding is usually restricted to the injection site, but occasionally stroke occurs. *Trials have shown that PCI (Chapter 16) is superior to lytic therapy when it can be done within 90 min after first medical contact.* **Streptokinase** is not an enzyme; it binds to circulating plasminogen to form an activator complex that converts further plasminogen to plasmin. Because there is a large excess of plasmin inhibitors in the blood, which can neutralize circulating plasmin, bleeding is not usually a problem. Within the thrombus the concentration of plasmin inhibitors is low, and so streptokinase has some selectivity for clots.

Alteplase is recombinant tissue-type plasminogen activator (rt-PA). Alteplase does not cause allergic reactions and can be used in patients when recent streptococcal infections or recent use of streptokinase contraindicates the use of streptokinase (i.e. patients in whom reperfusion may fail because of the action of neutralizing antibodies and who are at some risk of anaphylaxis). In contrast to streptokinase, coadministration of heparin with alteplase produces added benefit but increases the risk of stroke.

20 Lipid-lowering drugs

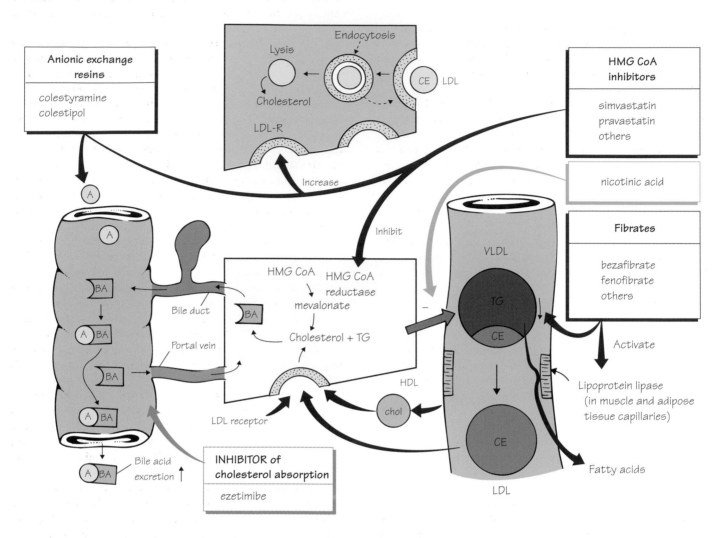

Lipids, such as triglycerides and cholesterylesters, are insoluble in water and are transported in plasma in the core of particles (**lipoproteins**) that have a hydrophilic shell of phospholipids and free cholesterol. This surface layer is stabilized by one or more **apolipoproteins**, which also act as ligands for cell surface **receptors**. About two-thirds of plasma lipoproteins are synthesized in the liver (middle, shaded (yellow)). Triglycerides (TG) are secreted into the blood as *very-low-density lipoproteins* (*VLDL*, ➡). In muscle and adipose tissue, the capillaries (right) possess an enzyme, *lipoprotein lipase* (▨), that hydrolyses the triglycerides to fatty acids; these then enter the muscle cells (for energy) and adipocytes (for storage). The residual particles containing a core rich in cholesterylester (CE) are called *low-density lipoprotein* (*LDL*) particles. The liver and other cells possess *LDL receptors* (⌒) that remove LDL from the plasma by endocytosis (top figure shaded orange). *The hepatic receptor-mediated removal of LDL is the main mechanism for controlling plasma LDL levels.*

Fatty acids and cholesterol from ingested dietary fat are re-esterified in mucosal cells of the intestine and form the core of *chylomicrons*, which enter the plasma via the thoracic duct. Fatty acids are hydrolysed

from the chylomicrons by lipoprotein lipase, and the residual triglyceride-depleted *remnants* are removed by the liver.

There is a strong positive correlation between the plasma concentration of LDL cholesterol and the development of **atherosclerosis** in medium and large arteries. Therapy that lowers LDL and raises high-density lipoprotein (HDL) has been shown to reduce the progression of coronary atherosclerosis. **Lipid-lowering drugs** are indicated most strongly in patients with coronary artery disease, or those with a high risk of coronary artery disease because of multiple risk factors, and in patients with familial hypercholesterolaemia. **Anion exchange resins** (top left, Ⓐ) bind bile acids (▯BA) and, because they are not absorbed, cholesterol excretion is increased. The **statins**, 3-hydroxy-3-methylglutaryl coenzyme A (**HMG CoA**) **reductase inhibitors** (top right), decrease hepatic cholesterol synthesis. The fall in hepatocyte cholesterol caused by resins and statins induces a compensatory increase in hepatic LDL receptors and consequently a fall in plasma cholesterol. **Nicotinic acid** (centre right) reduces the release of VLDL by the liver, whereas the **fibrates** (bottom right), which mainly lower triglyceride levels, probably act chiefly by stimulating lipoprotein lipase. **Ezetimibe** is the first of a new class of drugs that selectively inhibits the intestinal absorption of cholesterol.

Lipoproteins

These are classified according to their density on equilibrium ultracentrifugation. The larger particles (chylomicrons, remnants and VLDL) are the least dense and are not atherogenic because their greater size (diameter 30–500 nm) prevents them from passing into blood vessel walls. LDL particles (diameter 18–25 nm) can easily penetrate damaged arteries and are mainly responsible for the development of atherosclerosis. HDL particles are the smallest (diameter 5–12 nm), and epidemiological studies have revealed that high levels of HDL are associated with a lower incidence of atheroma. HDL accept excess (unesterified) cholesterol from cells and also from lipoproteins that have lost their triglycerides and therefore have an excess of surface components, including cholesterol. The cholesterol is made less polar by re-esterification, causing it to move into the hydrophobic core and leaving the surface available to accept more cholesterol. The cholesterylesters are then returned to the liver. The removal of cholesterol from artery walls by HDL is thought to be the basis of its antiatherogenic action.

Hyperlipidaemias

Primary lipoprotein disorders may involve cholesterol, triglycerides, or both. *Secondary* hyperlipidaemias are the result of another illness, e.g. diabetes mellitus or hypothyroidism. **Hypercholesterolaemia** is the most common disorder. About 5% of cases are familial but, in most cases, the cause is unknown. The main therapy for hyperlipidaemias, except for severe and hereditary types, is dietary modification (i.e. low fat and dietary restriction to obtain ideal body weight).

Atherosclerosis

It is not fully understood how atheromatous plaques develop in arteries, but turbulent flow is thought to initiate the process by causing focal damage to the intima. The plaques, which protrude into the lumen, are rich in cholesterol and have a lipid core covered by a fibrous cap. If the cap ruptures, the subintima acts as a focus for thrombosis, and occlusion of the artery may cause unstable angina, myocardial infarction or stroke. Epidemiological studies have shown a strong positive correlation between plasma cholesterol concentration (LDL) and coronary atherosclerosis, the incidence and severity of which is greatly increased by other risk factors, including cigarette smoking, hypertension, diabetes, family or personal history of premature heart disease, and left ventricular hypertrophy.

Lipid-lowering drugs

HMG CoA reductase inhibitors (statins) are the most important lipid-lowering drugs. They are very effective in lowering total and LDL cholesterol and have been shown to reduce coronary events and total mortality. They have few side-effects and are now usually the drugs of first choice. HMG CoA reductase inhibitors block the synthesis of cholesterol in the liver (which takes up most of the drug). This stimulates the expression of more enzyme, tending to restore cholesterol synthesis to normal even in the presence of the drug. However, this compensatory effect is incomplete and the reduction of cholesterol in the hepatocytes leads to an increased expression of LDL receptors, which increases the clearance of cholesterol from the plasma. Strong evidence that the statins lower plasma cholesterol, mainly by increasing the number of LDL receptors, is provided by the failure of the drugs to work in patients with homozygous familial hypercholesterolaemia (who have no LDL receptors).

Adverse effects are rare, the main one being myopathy. The incidence of myopathy is increased in patients given combined therapy with nicotinic acid or fibrates. Statins should not be given during pregnancy because cholesterol is essential for normal fetal development.

Anion exchange resins. Colestyramine and **colestipol** are powders taken with liquid. They increase the excretion of bile acids, causing more cholesterol to be converted to bile acids. The fall in hepatocyte cholesterol concentration causes compensatory increases in HMG CoA reductase activity and the number of LDL receptors. Because anion exchange resins do not work in patients with homozygous familial hypercholesterolaemia, it seems that increased expression of hepatic LDL receptors is the main mechanism by which resins lower plasma cholesterol.

Adverse effects are confined to the gut, because the resins are not absorbed; these effects include bloating, abdominal discomfort, diarrhoea and constipation.

Nicotinic acid reduces the release of VLDL and therefore lowers plasma triglycerides (by 30–50%). It also lowers cholesterol (by 10–20%) and increases HDL. Nicotinic acid was the first lipid-lowering drug to reduce overall mortality in patients with coronary artery disease, but its use is limited by unwanted effects, which include prostaglandin-mediated flushing, dizziness and palpitations. Nicotinic acid is now almost never used.

Fibrates (e.g. **gemfibrozil**, **bezafibrate**) produce a modest decrease in LDL (about 10%) and increase in HDL (about 10%). Moreover, they cause a marked fall in plasma triglycerides (about 30%). The fibrates act as ligands for the nuclear transcription receptor, peroxisome proliferator-activated receptor alpha (PPAR-α), and stimulate lipoprotein lipase activity. Fibrates are first-line drugs in patients with very high plasma triglyceride levels who are at risk of pancreatitis.

Adverse effects. All the fibrates can cause a myositis-like syndrome. The incidence of myositis is increased by concurrent use of HMG CoA inhibitors, and such combinations should be used with caution.

Inhibitors of intestinal cholesterol absorption. Ezetimibe reduces cholesterol (and phytosterol) absorption and decreases LDL cholesterol by about 18% with little change in HDL cholesterol. It may be synergistic with statins and is therefore a good choice for combination therapy.

Drug combinations

Severe hyperlipidaemia cannot always be controlled with a single drug, and combination therapy is increasingly being used to achieve target lipid levels. Combinations should involve drugs with different mechanisms of action, e.g. a statin with a fibrate. Although the combination of statins with fibrates (and nicotinic acid) may increase the incidence of myopathy, it is increasingly believed that the benefit of lowering LDL cholesterol in these patients outweighs the small increase in the risk of adverse effects. Interest in fibrates has been increased by a recent trial showing that gemfibrozil reduced myocardial infarction, stroke and overall mortality in men with coronary artery disease associated with low HDL cholesterol. The drug increased HDL cholesterol without decreasing LDL cholesterol.

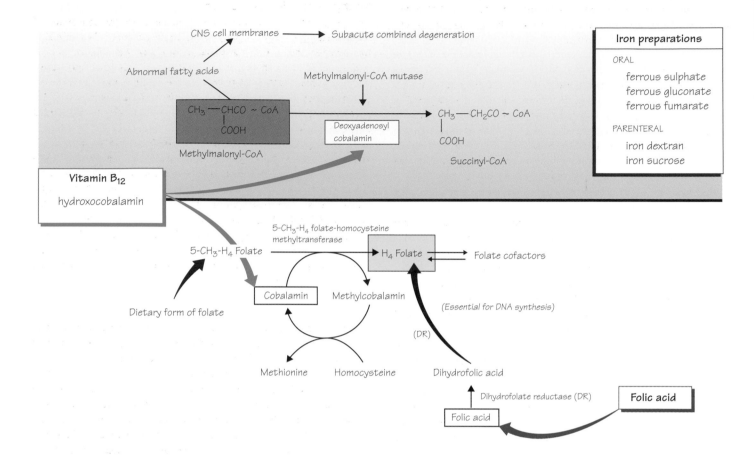

Normal erythropoiesis requires iron, vitamin B_{12} and folic acid. A deficiency of any of these causes anaemia. Erythropoietic activity is regulated by **erythropoietin**, a hormone released mainly by the kidneys. In chronic renal failure, anaemia often occurs because of a fall in erythropoietin production.

Iron is necessary for haemoglobin production, and iron deficiency results in small red blood cells with insufficient haemoglobin (microcytic hypochromic anaemia). The administration of iron preparations (top right) is needed in iron deficiency, which may be because of chronic blood loss (e.g. menorrhagia), pregnancy (the fetus takes iron from the mother), various abnormalities of the gut (iron absorption may be reduced) or premature birth (such babies are born with very low iron stores).

The main problem with oral iron preparations is that they frequently cause *gastrointestinal upsets*. Oral therapy is continued until haemoglobin is normal and the body stores of iron are built up by several months of lower iron doses. Children are very sensitive to iron toxicity and can be killed by as little as 1 g of ferrous sulphate. Overdosage of iron is treated with oral and parenteral **desferrioxamine**, a potent iron-chelating agent.

Vitamin B_{12} and **folic acid** are essential for several reactions necessary for normal DNA synthesis. A deficiency of either vitamin causes impaired production and abnormal maturation of erythroid precursor cells (megaloblastic anaemia). In addition to anaemia, vitamin B_{12} deficiency causes *central nervous system degeneration* (subacute combined degeneration), which may result in psychiatric or physical symptoms. The anaemia is caused by a block of H_4 folate synthesis (lower figure, ▢) and the nervous degeneration is caused by an accumulation of methylmalonyl-CoA (upper figure, ▨).

Vitamin B_{12} deficiency occurs when there is malabsorption because of a lack of intrinsic factor (pernicious anaemia), following gastrectomy (no intrinsic factor), or in various small bowel diseases in which absorption is impaired. Because the disease is nearly always caused by malabsorption, oral vitamin administration is of little value, and replacement therapy, usually for life, involves injections of vitamin B_{12} (left). **Hydroxocobalamin** is the form of choice for therapy because it is retained in the body longer than cyanocobalamin (cyanocobalamin is bound less to plasma proteins and is more rapidly excreted in urine).

Folic acid deficiency leading to a megaloblastic anaemia, which requires oral folic acid (bottom right), may occur in pregnancy (folate requirement is increased) and in malabsorption syndromes (e.g. steatorrhoea and sprue).

Neutropenia caused by anticancer drugs can be shortened in duration by treatment with recombinant human granulocyte colony-stimulating factor (**lenograstim**). Although the incidence of sepsis may be reduced, there is no evidence that the drug improves overall survival.

Iron

The nucleus of haem is formed by iron, which, in combination with the appropriate globin chains, forms the protein haemoglobin. Over 90% of the non-storage iron in the body is in haemoglobin (about 2.3 g). Some iron (about 1 g) is stored as ferritin and haemosiderin in macrophages in the spleen, liver and bone marrow.

Absorption

Iron is normally absorbed in the duodenum and proximal jejunum. Normally 5–10% of dietary iron is absorbed (about 0.5–1 mg day^{-1}), but this can be increased if iron stores are low. Iron must be in the ferrous form for absorption, which occurs by active transport. In the plasma, iron is transported bound to transferrin, a β-globulin. There is no mechanism for the excretion of iron, and the regulation of iron balance is achieved by appropriate changes in iron absorption.

Iron preparations

For oral therapy, iron preparations contain ferrous salts because these are absorbed most efficiently. In iron-deficient patients, about 50–100 mg of iron can be incorporated into haemoglobin daily. Because about 25% of oral ferrous salts can be absorbed, 100–200 mg of iron should be given daily for the fastest possible correction of deficiency. If this causes intolerable gastrointestinal irritation (nausea, epigastric pain, diarrhoea, constipation), lower doses can be given; these will completely correct the iron deficiency, but more slowly.

Parenteral iron does not hasten the haemoglobin response and should only be used if oral therapy has failed as a result of continuing severe blood loss, malabsorption or lack of patient cooperation.

Iron dextran is a complex of ferric hydroxide with dextrans. **Iron sucrose** is a complex of ferric hydroxide with sucrose. These drugs are given by intravenous injection or infusion. Severe reactions may occur, and drugs for resuscitation and anaphylaxis should be available.

Iron toxicity

Acute toxicity occurs most commonly in young children who have ingested iron tablets. These cause necrotizing gastroenteritis with abdominal pain, vomiting, bloody diarrhoea and, later, shock. This may be followed, even after apparent improvement, by acidosis, coma and death.

Vitamin B$_{12}$

In megaloblastic anaemias, the underlying defect is impaired DNA synthesis. Cell division is decreased but RNA and protein synthesis continue. This results in large (macrocytic), fragile red cells. The cobalt atom at the centre of the vitamin B$_{12}$ molecule covalently binds different ligands, forming various cobalamins. *Methylcobalamin* and *deoxyadenosylcobalamin* are the active forms of the vitamin, and other cobalamins must be converted to these active forms.

Vitamin B$_{12}$ (extrinsic factor) is absorbed only when complexed with *intrinsic factor*, a glycoprotein secreted by the *parietal cells* of the gastric mucosa. Absorption occurs in the distal ileum by a highly specific transport process, and the vitamin is then transported bound to transcobalamin II (a plasma glycoprotein). *Pernicious anaemia* results from a *deficiency* in intrinsic factor caused by autoantibodies, either to the factor itself or to the gastric parietal cells (atrophic gastritis).

Methylmalonyl-CoA mutase

This enzyme requires deoxyadenosylcobalamin for the conversion of methylmalonyl-CoA to succinyl-CoA. In the absence of vitamin B$_{12}$, this reaction cannot take place and there is accumulation of *methylmalonyl-CoA*. This results in the synthesis of abnormal fatty acids, which become incorporated in neuronal membranes and may cause the neurological defects seen in vitamin B$_{12}$ deficiency. However, it is also possible that the disruption of methionine synthesis may be involved in the neuronal damage.

5-CH$_3$-H$_4$ folate-homocysteine methyltransferase converts 5-CH$_3$-H$_4$ folate and homocysteine to H$_4$ folate and methionine. In this reaction, cobalamin is converted to methylcobalamin. When vitamin B$_{12}$ deficiency prevents this reaction, the conversion of the major dietary and storage folate (5-CH$_3$-H$_4$ folate) to the precursor of folate cofactors (H$_4$ folate) cannot occur and a deficiency in the folate cofactors necessary for DNA synthesis develops. This reaction links folic acid and vitamin B$_{12}$ metabolism and explains why high doses of folic acid can improve the anaemia, but not the nervous degeneration, caused by vitamin B$_{12}$ deficiency.

Folic acid

The body stores of folates are relatively low (5–20 mg) and, as daily requirements are high, folic acid deficiency and megaloblastic anaemia can quickly develop (1–6 months) if the intake of folic acid stops. Folic acid itself is completely absorbed in the proximal jejunum, but dietary folates are mainly polyglutamate forms of 5-CH$_3$-H$_4$ folate. All but one of the glutamyl residues are hydrolysed off before the absorption of monoglutamate 5-CH$_3$-H$_4$ folate. In contrast to vitamin B$_{12}$ deficiency, folic acid deficiency is often caused by inadequate dietary intake of folate. Some drugs (e.g. *phenytoin*, *oral contraceptives*, *isoniazid*) can cause folic acid deficiency by reducing its absorption.

Folic acid and vitamin B$_{12}$ have no known toxic effects. However, it is important not to give folic acid alone in vitamin B$_{12}$ deficiency states because, although the anaemia may improve, the neurological degeneration progresses and may become irreversible.

Erythropoietin

Hypoxia, or loss of blood, results in increased haemoglobin synthesis and the release of erythrocytes. These changes are mediated by an increase in circulating erythropoietin (a glycoprotein containing 166 amino acid residues). Erythropoietin binds to receptors on erythroid cell precursors in the bone marrow and increases the transcription of enzymes involved in haem synthesis. Recombinant human erythropoietin is available as **epoetin alfa** and **epoetin beta**, the two forms being clinically indistinguishable. **Darbepoetin alfa** is a glycosylated derivative of epoetin alfa and, because it has a longer half-life, it can be given less frequently than epoetin alfa. These recombinant erythropoietins are given by intravenous or subcutaneous injection to correct anaemia in chronic renal failure disease – such anaemia is caused largely by a deficiency of the hormone. Epoetin is also used to treat anaemia caused by platinum-containing anticancer drugs.

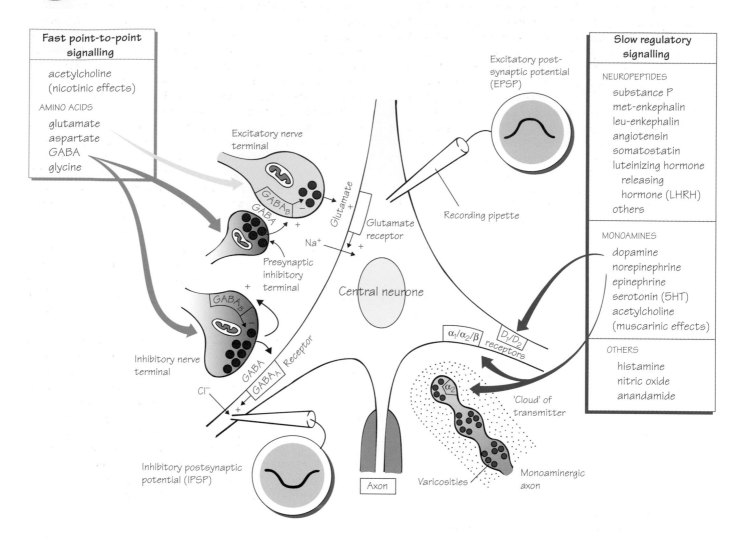

Fast point-to-point signalling

acetylcholine (nicotinic effects)

AMINO ACIDS
glutamate
aspartate
GABA
glycine

Slow regulatory signalling

NEUROPEPTIDES
substance P
met-enkephalin
leu-enkephalin
angiotensin
somatostatin
luteinizing hormone releasing hormone (LHRH)
others

MONOAMINES
dopamine
norepinephrine
epinephrine
serotonin (5HT)
acetylcholine (muscarinic effects)

OTHERS
histamine
nitric oxide
anandamide

Excitatory post-synaptic potential (EPSP)

Recording pipette

Excitatory nerve terminal

Presynaptic inhibitory terminal

Glutamate receptor

Central neurone

Inhibitory nerve terminal

GABA Receptor

Inhibitory postsynaptic potential (IPSP)

Axon

Varicosities

'Cloud' of transmitter

Monoaminergic axon

$\alpha_1/\alpha_2/\beta$ D_1/D_2 receptors

Drugs acting on the central nervous system are used more than any other type of agent. In addition to their therapeutic uses, drugs such as **caffeine, alcohol** and **nicotine** are used socially to provide a sense of well-being. Central drugs often produce dependence with continued use (Chapter 31), and many are subject to strict legal controls.

The mechanisms by which central drugs produce their therapeutic effects are usually unknown, reflecting our lack of understanding of neurological and psychiatric disease. Knowledge of central transmitter substances is important because virtually all drugs acting on the brain produce their effects by modifying synaptic transmission.

The transmitters used in fast point-to-point neural circuits are **amino acids** (left), except for a few cholinergic synapses with nicotinic receptors. **Glutamate** is the main central excitatory transmitter. It depolarizes neurones by triggering an increase in membrane Na^+ conductance. **γ-Aminobutyric acid (GABA)** is the main inhibitory transmitter, being released at perhaps one-third of all central synapses. It hyperpolarizes neurones by increasing their membrane Cl^- conductance and stabilizes

the resting membrane potential near the Cl^- equilibrium potential. **Glycine** is also an inhibitory transmitter, mainly in the spinal cord.

In addition to fast point-to-point signalling, the brain possesses more diffuse regulatory systems, which use **monoamines** as their transmitters (middle right). The cell bodies of these branched axons project to many areas of the brain. Transmitter release occurs diffusely from many points along varicose terminal networks of monoaminergic neurones, affecting very large numbers of target cells. The functions of the central monoaminergic pathways are not fully understood, but they are involved in disorders such as *Parkinson's disease, depression, migraine* and *schizophrenia*.

Over 40 **peptides** (top right) have been found in central neurones and nerve terminals. The evidence for their role as transmitter substances is usually very incomplete. They form another group of diffusely acting regulatory transmitters, but as yet the physiological roles of many of them are unknown.

Other substances that are thought to be central transmitters include nitric oxide, histamine and anandamide (bottom right).

Amino acids

γ-Aminobutyric acid is present in all areas of the central nervous system, mainly in local inhibitory interneurones. It rapidly inhibits central neurones, the response being mediated by postsynaptic $GABA_A$ receptors, which are blocked by the convulsant drug bicuculline. Some GABA receptors ($GABA_B$) are not blocked by bicuculline, but are selectively activated by **baclofen** (*p*-chlorophenyl-GABA). Many $GABA_B$ receptors are located on presynaptic nerve terminals, and their activation results in a reduction in transmitter release (e.g. of glutamate and GABA itself). Baclofen reduces glutamate release in the spinal cord and produces an antispastic effect, which is useful in controlling the muscular spasms that occur in diseases such as multiple sclerosis.

Following their release from presynaptic nerve terminals, amino acid transmitters are inactivated by reuptake systems.

Drugs that are thought to act by modifying GABAergic synaptic transmission include the **benzodiazepines**, **barbiturates** (Chapter 24) and the anticonvulsants **vigabatrin** and perhaps **valproate** (Chapter 25).

Glycine is an inhibitory transmitter in spinal interneurones. It is antagonized by strychnine and its release is prevented by tetanus toxin, both substances causing convulsions.

Glutamate excites virtually all central neurones by activating several types of excitatory amino acid receptor. These receptors are classified into (ligand-gated) kainate, AMPA (α-amino-3-hydroxy-5-methyl-4-isoxazolepropionic acid) and NMDA (*N*-methyl-D-aspartate) receptors, depending on whether or not they are selectively activated by these glutamate analogues. A family of metabotropic (G-protein-coupled) receptors also exists. NMDA receptor antagonists (e.g. 2-aminophosphonovalerate) have been shown to have anticonvulsant activity in many experimental animal models of epilepsy, and they may prove to be beneficial in stroke, where at least some of the neuronal damage is thought to result from excessive release of glutamate. Lamotrigine is an antiepileptic drug (Chapter 25) that is thought to act partly by reducing presynaptic glutamate release.

Monoamines

Acetylcholine is mainly excitatory in the brain. It is the transmitter released from motor neurone nerve endings at the neuromuscular junction and at collateral axon synapses with Renshaw cells in the spinal cord. The excitatory effects of acetylcholine on central neurones are usually mediated via muscarinic receptors, predominantly of the M_1 subtype. Nicotinic receptors are also present in the brain. They have a different subunit construction (e.g. $\alpha_4\beta_2$) from peripheral receptors and a different pharmacology. Most central nicotinic receptors are presynaptic and increase the release of many other transmitters. However, their only known clinical importance is in nicotine dependence (Chapter 31).

Cholinergic neurones are particularly abundant in the basal ganglia and others seem to be involved in cortical arousal responses and in memory. **Atropine-like** drugs can impair memory, and the amnesic action of **hyoscine** is exploited in anaesthetic premedication (Chapter 23). They are also used for their central actions in *motion sickness* (Chapter 30) and *Parkinson's disease* (Chapter 26). Loss of cholinergic neurones and memory are prominent features of *Alzheimer's disease*, a common form of senile dementia for which there is no effective treatment at present. **Donepezil** and **rivastigmine** are anticholinesterases of modest benefit in up to 50% of patients with Alzheimer's disease.

Dopamine generally inhibits central neurones by opening K^+ channels. Dopaminergic pathways project from the *substantia nigra* in the midbrain to the basal ganglia and from the *midbrain* to the limbic cortex and other limbic structures. A third (tuberoinfundibular) pathway is involved in regulating prolactin release. The nigrostriatal pathway is concerned with modulating the control of voluntary movement and its degeneration results in *Parkinson's disease*. The mesolimbic pathway is 'overactive' in *schizophrenia*, but it is not known why. Dopamine *agonists* are used in the treatment of Parkinson's disease (Chapter 26) and *antagonists* (neuroleptics) are used in schizophrenia (Chapter 27). The chemoreceptor trigger zone (CTZ) has dopamine receptors, and dopamine antagonists have *antiemetic* effects (Chapter 30).

Norepinephrine both inhibits and excites central neurones by activating α_2- and α_1/β-receptors, respectively. Norepinephrine-containing cell bodies occur in several groups in the brainstem. The largest of these nuclei is the *locus coeruleus* in the pons, which projects to the entire dorsal forebrain, especially the cerebral cortex and hippocampus. The hypothalamus also possesses a high density of noradrenergic fibres. Norepinephrine and dopamine in limbic forebrain structures (especially the nucleus accumbens) may be involved in an ascending 'reward' system, which has been implicated in *drug dependence* (Chapter 31). Ascending noradrenergic pathways are also involved in arousal, especially in response to unfamiliar or threatening stimuli. Depressed patients are often unresponsive to external stimuli (low arousal) and impairment of noradrenergic function may be associated with *depression* (Chapter 28). Norepinephrine in the medulla is involved in blood pressure regulation (Chapter 15).

Serotonin (5-hydroxytryptamine, 5HT) occurs in cell bodies in the *raphe nucleus* of the brainstem, which projects to many forebrain areas and to the ventral and dorsal horns of the spinal cord. The latter descending projection modulates pain inputs (Chapter 29). 5HT pathways are involved in feeding behaviour, sleep and mood. 5HT may, like norepinephrine, be involved in *depression*. $5HT_3$ receptors occur in the CTZ, and antagonists have antiemetic effects. $5HT_{1D}$ receptors occur in cranial blood vessels, and the agonist **sumatriptan** relieves migraine by constricting the vessels that are abnormally dilated during the attack. 5HT is involved in the control of sensory transmission, and $5HT_2$ agonists (e.g. **LSD**) cause hallucinations (Chapter 31).

Other transmitters/modulaters

Histamine is a relatively minor transmitter in the brain, but H_1 receptor-antagonists cause sedation and have antiemetic actions (Chapter 30).

Neuropeptides form the most numerous group of possible central transmitters, but little is known yet of their functions. Substance P and the enkephalins are involved in pain pathways (Chapter 29).

Nitric oxide (**NO**). Nitric oxide synthase (NOS) is present in about 1–2% of neurones in many areas of the brain, e.g. cerebral cortex, hippocampus, striatum. NO has been shown to have many actions in the brain and it is believed to have a modulatory role. It affects the release of other transmitters and there is evidence that it may be involved in synaptic plasticity, e.g. long-term potentiation. No therapeutic agents are known to involve central NO but important drugs acting via NO are **organic vasodilators** used in angina (Chapter 16) and **phosphodiesterase-5 inhibitors** used in erectile dysfunction (Chapter 7).

Anandamide acts at cannabinoid CB1 receptors and is termed an **endocannabinoid**. The role of anandamide is unknown. However, CB1 receptors are involved in the actions of Δ^9-tetrahydrocannabinol (THC), the active constituent of cannabis (Chapter 31), and apparently in food intake, because the CB_1-receptor antagonist **rimonabant** causes a modest (5%) loss of weight in obese patients. Unfortunately, recent evidence indicates that rimonabant is associated with an increased incidence of anxiety and depression.

23 General anaesthetics

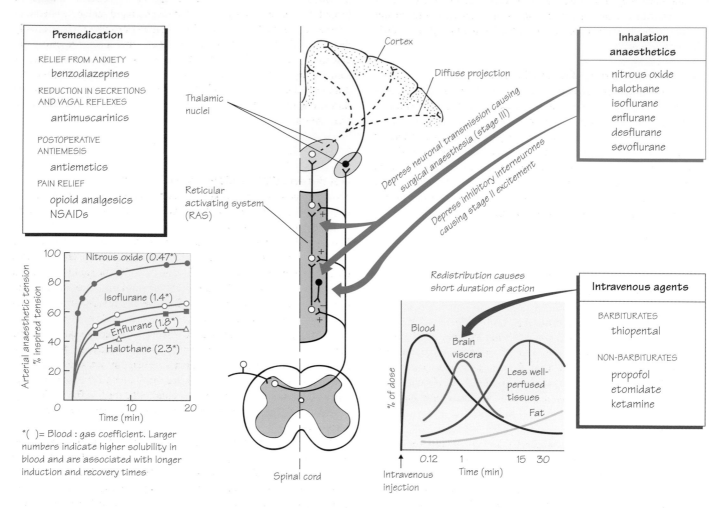

*( )= Blood : gas coefficient. Larger numbers indicate higher solubility in blood and are associated with longer induction and recovery times

General anaesthesia is the absence of sensation associated with a reversible loss of consciousness. Numerous agents ranging from inert gases to steroids produce anaesthesia in animals, but only a few are used clinically (right). Historical anaesthetics include ether, chloroform, cyclopropane, ethylchloride and trichlorethylene.

Anaesthetics depress all excitable tissues including central neurones, cardiac muscle, and smooth and striatal muscle. However, these tissues have different sensitivities to anaesthetics, and the areas of the brain responsible for consciousness (middle, ▨) are among the most sensitive. Thus, it is possible to administer anaesthetic agents at concentrations that produce unconsciousness without unduly depressing the cardiovascular and respiratory centres or the myocardium. However, for most anaesthetics, *the margin of safety is small*.

General anaesthesia usually involves the administration of different drugs for:
- **premedication** (top left);
- **induction** of anaesthesia (bottom right); and
- **maintenance** of anaesthesia (top right).

Premedication has two main aims:

1 the prevention of the parasympathomimetic effects of anaesthesia (bradycardia, bronchial secretion); and

2 the reduction of anxiety or pain.

Premedication is often omitted for minor operations. If necessary, the appropriate drugs (e.g. hyoscine) are given intravenously at induction.

Induction is most commonly achieved by the intravenous injection of **propofol** or **thiopental**. Unconsciousness occurs within seconds and is maintained by the administration of an inhalation anaesthetic. **Halothane** was the first fluorinated volatile anaesthetic and was widely used in the UK. However, it is associated with a very low incidence of potentially fatal hepatotoxicity and has largely been replaced with newer, less toxic agents, e.g. **sevoflurane** and **isoflurane**. **Nitrous oxide** at concentrations up to 70% in oxygen is the most widely used anaesthetic agent. It is used with oxygen as a carrier gas for the volatile agents, or together with opioid analgesics (e.g. *fentanyl*). Nitrous oxide causes sedation and analgesia, but it is not sufficient alone to maintain anaesthesia.

During the induction of anaesthesia, distinct 'stages' occur with some agents, especially ether. First, analgesia is produced (stage I), followed by excitement (stage II) caused by inhibition of inhibitory reticular neurones (●—◖). Then surgical anaesthesia (stage III) develops, the depth of which depends on the amount of drug administered. These stages are not obvious with currently used anaesthetics.

Reticular activating system (RAS)

This is a complex polysynaptic pathway in the brainstem reticular formation that projects diffusely to the cortex. Activity in the RAS is concerned with maintaining consciousness and, because it is especially sensitive to the depressant action of anaesthetics, it is thought to be their primary site of action.

Mechanism of action of anaesthetics

It is not known how anaesthetics produce their effects. Because anaesthetic potency correlates well with lipid solubility it was thought that anaesthetics might dissolve in the lipid bilayer of the cell membrane and somehow produce anaesthesia by expanding the membrane or increasing its fluidity. It is now believed that anaesthetics bind to a hydrophobic area of a protein (e.g. ion channel, receptor) and inhibit its normal function. In support of this idea, anaesthetics have been shown to inhibit the function of glutamate receptors and to enhance γ-aminobutyric acid (GABA)ergic transmission.

Premedication

Relief from anxiety (see Chapter 24)

Oral **benzodiazepines**, such as lorazepam, are most effective.

Reduction of secretions and vagal reflexes

Antimuscarinics, usually **hyoscine**, are no longer used routinely for premedication. They prevent salivation and bronchial secretions and, more importantly, protect the heart from arrhythmias, particularly bradycardia caused by halothane, propofol, suxamethonium and neostigmine. Hyoscine is also antiemetic and produces some amnesia.

Analgesics

Opioid analgesics, e.g. morphine (Chapter 29), are rarely given before an operation unless the patient is in pain. **Fentanyl** and related drugs (e.g. **alfentanyl**) are used intravenously to supplement nitrous oxide anaesthesia. These opioids are highly lipid soluble and have a rapid onset of action. They have a short duration of action because of redistribution. **Non-steroidal anti-inflammatory drugs** (**NSAIDs**) (e.g. **diclofenac**) may provide sufficient postoperative analgesia and do not cause respiratory depression. They can be given orally or by injection.

Postoperative antiemesis

Nausea and vomiting are very common after anaesthesia. Often, opioid drugs given during and after the operation are responsible. Sometimes antiemetic drugs are given with the premedication, but they are more effective if administered intravenously during anaesthesia. The dopamine antagonist **droperidol** is widely used for this purpose and is effective against opioid-induced emesis.

Intravenous agents

These are used mainly for the induction of anaesthesia. Some agents, particularly propofol, are used alone (by continuous infusion) for short surgical procedures.

Thiopental injected intravenously induces anaesthesia in less than 30 s because the very lipid-soluble drug quickly dissolves in the rapidly perfused brain. Recovery from a single dose of thiopental is also rapid because of redistribution into less well-perfused tissues (bottom right figure). The liver subsequently metabolizes thiopental. Doses of thiopental only slightly above the 'sleep dose' depress the myocardium and the respiratory centre. Very occasionally anaphylaxis may occur.

Propofol (2,6-diisopropylphenol) induces anaesthesia within 30 s and is smooth and pleasant. Recovery from propofol is rapid without nausea or hangover and, for this reason, it has largely replaced thiopental. Propofol is inactivated by redistribution and rapid metabolism and, in contrast to thiopental, recovery from continuous infusion is relatively fast. **Etomidate** is an unpleasant anaesthetic that is sometimes used in emergency anaesthesia because it causes less cardiovascular depression and hypotension than other agents. **Ketamine** may be given by intramuscular or intravenous injection. It is analgesic in subanaesthetic doses, but often causes hallucinations. Its main use is in paediatric anaesthesia.

Inhalation agents

Uptake and distribution (bottom left figure)

The speed at which induction of anaesthesia occurs depends mainly on the *solubility of gas in blood* and the *inspired concentration of gas*. When agents of low solubility (nitrous oxide) diffuse from the lungs into arterial blood, relatively small amounts are required to saturate the blood, and so the arterial tension (and hence brain tension) rises quickly. More soluble agents (halothane) require the solution of much more anaesthetic before the arterial anaesthetic tension approaches that of the inspired gas and so induction is slower. Recovery from anaesthesia is also slower with increasing anaesthetic solubility.

Nitrous oxide is not potent enough to use as a sole anaesthetic agent, but it is commonly used as a non-flammable carrier gas for volatile agents, allowing their concentration to be significantly reduced. It is a good analgesic, and a 50% mixture in oxygen (Entonox) is used when analgesia is required (e.g. in childbirth, road traffic accidents). Nitrous oxide has little effect on the cardiovascular or respiratory systems.

Halothane is a potent agent and, as the vapour is non-irritant, induction is smooth and pleasant. It causes a concentration-dependent hypotension, largely by myocardial depression. Halothane often causes arrhythmias and, because the myocardium is sensitized to catecholamines, infiltration of epinephrine (adrenaline) may cause cardiac arrest. Like most volatile anaesthetics, halothane depresses the respiratory centre. More than 20% of the administered halothane is biotransformed by the liver to metabolites (e.g. trifluoroacetic acid) that may cause severe hepatotoxicity with a high mortality. Hepatotoxicity is more likely after repeated exposure to halothane, which should be avoided.

Isoflurane has similar actions to halothane, but is less cardiodepressant and does not sensitize the heart to epinephrine. It causes dose-related hypotension by decreasing systemic vascular resistance. Only 0.2% of the absorbed dose is metabolized and none of the metabolites has been associated with hepatotoxicity.

Sevoflurane has a low blood-to-gas coefficient (0.6), and emergence and recovery from anaesthesia are rapid. This may necessitate early postoperative pain relief. It is very pleasant to breathe, and is a good choice if an inhalation agent is required for induction, e.g. in children.

Enflurane is similar in action to halothane. It undergoes much less metabolism (2%) than halothane and is unlikely to cause hepatotoxicity. The disadvantage of enflurane is that it may cause seizure activity and, occasionally, muscle twitching.

Desflurane is similar to isoflurane, but less potent. Because higher concentrations must be inhaled, it may cause respiratory tract irritation (cough, breath-holding). Desflurane has low blood solubility (blood-to-gas ratio = 0.4) and so recovery is rapid.

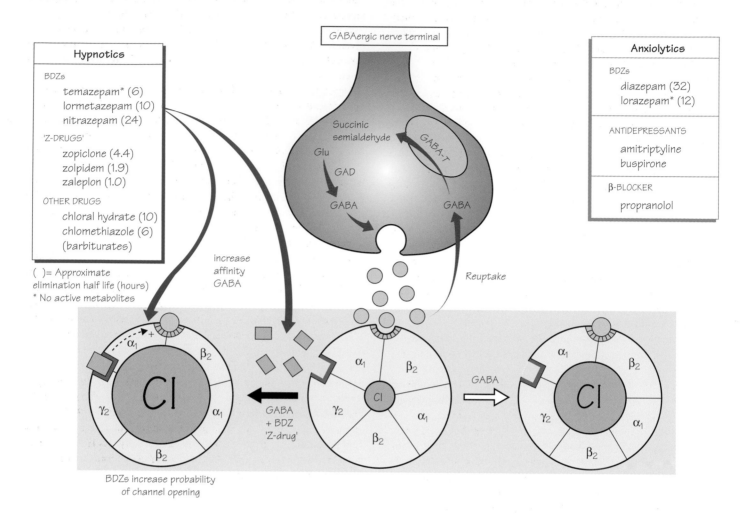

Hypnotics

BDZs
  temazepam* (6)
  lormetazepam (10)
  nitrazepam (24)

'Z-DRUGS'
  zopiclone (4.4)
  zolpidem (1.9)
  zaleplon (1.0)

OTHER DRUGS
  chloral hydrate (10)
  chlomethiazole (6)
  (barbiturates)

( )= Approximate
elimination half life (hours)
* No active metabolites

Anxiolytics

BDZs
  diazepam (32)
  lorazepam* (12)

ANTIDEPRESSANTS
  amitriptyline
  buspirone

β-BLOCKER
  propranolol

GABAergic nerve terminal

Succinic semialdehyde
Glu
GAD
GABA
GABA-T
GABA

increase affinity GABA

Reuptake

GABA + BDZ 'Z-drug'

GABA

BDZs increase probability of channel opening

Drug treatment of *sleep disorders* (hypnotics) and *acute anxiety states* (anxiolytics) is dominated by the **benzodiazepines** (BDZs). In general, these drugs will induce sleep when given in high doses at night and will provide sedation and reduce anxiety when given in low, divided doses during the day.

BDZs have *anxiolytic, hypnotic, muscle relaxant, anticonvulsant* (Chapter 25) and *amnesic* actions, which are thought to be caused mainly by the enhancement of *γ-aminobutyric acid (GABA)-mediated inhibition* in the central nervous system. GABA (⚪) released from nerve terminals (top middle, shaded) binds to **GABA$_A$ receptors** (⚓); the activation of these receptors increases the Cl$^-$ conductance of the neurone (bottom right). The GABA$_A$–Cl$^-$ channel complex also has a BDZ modulatory receptor site (⊔). Occupation of the BDZ sites by BDZ receptor agonists (▢) causes a conformational change in the GABA receptor. This increases the affinity of GABA binding and enhances the actions of GABA on the Cl$^-$ conductance of the neuronal membrane (bottom left). The **barbiturates** act at another binding site and similarly enhance the action of GABA (not illustrated). In the absence of GABA, BDZs and low doses of barbiturates do not affect Cl$^-$ conductance.

The popularity of BDZs arose from their apparently low toxicity, but it is now realized that chronic BDZ treatment may cause cognitive

impairment, tolerance and **dependence**. For these reasons, BDZs should only be used for 2–4 weeks to treat severe anxiety and insomnia.

Many **antidepressants** (e.g. **amitriptyline**) are also anxiolytic and do not cause dependence. **Buspirone** is a non-sedative anxiolytic that acts at 5-hydroxytryptamine (5HT) synapses. **β-Blockers** can be useful in anxiety where autonomic symptoms predominate (e.g. tremor, tachycardia, sweating).

Different BDZs are marketed as hypnotics (top left) and anxiolytics (top right). It is mainly the duration of action that determines the choice of drug. Many BDZs are metabolized in the liver to **active metabolites**, which may have longer elimination half-lives ($t_{1/2}$) than the parent drug. For example, **diazepam** ($t_{1/2} \approx 20–80$ h) has an active *N*-desmethyl metabolite that has an elimination half-life of up to 200 h.

BDZs used as hypnotics (top left) can be divided into short-acting and longer-acting. A rapidly eliminated drug (e.g. **temazepam**) is usually preferred to avoid daytime sedation. A longer-acting drug (e.g. **lormetazepam**) may be preferred where early morning waking is a problem and where a daytime anxiolytic effect is needed. **Zopiclone, zolpidem** and **zaleplon** are not BZDs but act at BDZ receptors. They have short durations of action and because they are likely to cause less daytime sedation are increasingly popular as hypnotics.

GABA receptors

GABA receptors (Chapter 22) of the $GABA_A$ type are involved in the actions of hypnotics/anxiolytics. The $GABA_A$ receptor belongs to the superfamily of ligand-gated ion channels (other examples are the nicotinic, glycine and $5HT_3$ receptors). The $GABA_A$ receptor consists of five subunits (bottom figure). Variants of each of these subunits have been cloned (six α-, four β-, three γ- and one δ-subunit). Several other subunits exist, but it seems that most $GABA_A$ receptors comprise two α-, two β- and one γ-subunit. A major type is probably $2\alpha_1$, $2\beta_2$, γ_2 because mRNAs encoding these subunits are often co-localized in the brain. Electrophysiological experiments on toad oocytes possessing various combinations of $GABA_A$ subunits (produced by injecting their mRNA into the oocyte) have revealed that receptors constructed from α- and β-subunits respond to GABA (i.e. the Cl^- conductance increases), but for a receptor to respond fully to a BDZ, a γ_2-subunit is required. In mice, it seems that the α_1-subunit is involved, particularly in the sedative action of BDZs, because a point mutation in the α_1-subunit (arginine replaces histidine at position 101) results in transgenic mice that are resistant to the sedative (and amnesic) effect of diazepam without affecting its anxiolytic action. In contrast, similar mutations in the α_2-subunit of GABA receptors result in mice that are resistant to the anxiolytic effect of BDZs. These studies suggest that $GABA_A$ receptors containing the α_2-subunit are involved in the anxiolytic action of BDZs, whereas receptors containing the α_1-subunit are involved in the sedative actions of BDZs. However, it remains to be seen whether a non-sedative, subunit-selective drug can be found to reduce anxiety in humans.

Some drugs that bind to the BDZ receptor actually increase anxiety and are called **inverse agonists**. In the absence of ligand, most receptors are believed to be in a resting state (Chapter 2), but BDZ receptors are appreciably activated, even when no ligand is present. Inverse agonists are anxiogenic because they convert activated BDZ receptors to the resting state. Antagonists do the same thing, and this may explain why BDZ antagonists (e.g. **flumazenil**) are sometimes anxiogenic and very rarely cause convulsions, particularly in epileptics.

Flumazenil is a competitive BDZ antagonist that has a short duration of action and is given intravenously. It can be used to reverse the sedative effects of BDZs in anaesthesia, intensive care, diagnostic procedures and in overdoses.

Barbiturate receptor

Barbiturates (and chloral hydrate and chlormethiazole) are far more depressant than BDZs, because at higher doses they increase the Cl^- conductance directly and decrease the sensitivity of the neuronal postsynaptic membrane to excitatory transmitters.

Barbiturates were extensively used but are now obsolete as hypnotics and anxiolytics because they readily lead to psychological and physical dependence, they induce microsomal enzymes, and relatively small overdosages may be fatal. In contrast, huge overdoses of BDZs have been taken without serious long-term effects. Barbiturates (e.g. **thiopental**, Chapter 23) retain a role in anaesthesia and are still used as anticonvulsants (e.g. **phenobarbital**, Chapter 25).

Benzodiazepines (BDZs)

These are active orally and, although most are metabolized by oxidation in the liver, they do not induce hepatic enzyme systems. They are central depressants but, in contrast to other hypnotics and anxiolytics, their maximum effect when given orally does not normally cause fatal, or even severe, respiratory depression. However, respiratory depression may occur in patients with bronchopulmonary disease or with intravenous administration. **Adverse effects** include drowsiness, impaired alertness, agitation and ataxia, especially in the elderly.

Dependence. A physical withdrawal syndrome may occur in patients given BDZs for even short periods. The symptoms, which may persist for weeks or months, include anxiety, insomnia, depression, nausea and perceptual changes.

Drug interactions. BDZs have additive or synergistic effects with other central depressants such as alcohol, barbiturates and antihistamines.

Intravenous BDZs (e.g. **diazepam**, **lorazepam**) are used in status epilepticus (Chapter 25) and very occasionally in panic attacks (however, oral **alprazolam** is probably more effective for this latter purpose and is safer). **Midazolam**, unlike other BDZs, forms water-soluble salts and is used as an intravenous sedative during endoscopic and dental procedures. When given intravenously, BDZs have an *impressive amnesic action* and patients may remember nothing of unpleasant procedures. Intravenous BDZs may cause respiratory depression, and assisted ventilation may be required.

Zopiclone, zolpidem and zaleplon, so called Z-drugs, have shorter half-lives than the BDZs. Mouse mutation studies have shown that zolpidem and zaleplon have a selective action on the α_1-subunit. They all have reduced propensity to tolerance and have less abuse liability. Zaleplon has such a short half-life that it can be used to treat middle-of-night insomnia as long as a 5-h period elapses before driving, etc.

Antidepressants

Tricyclic antidepressants, such as **amitriptyline**, have anxiolytic effects. They are used in patients with depression and anxiety, and for patients who require long-term anxiolytic drugs where BDZs would result in dependence. Monoamine oxidase inhibitors, e.g. **moclobemide**, may be especially useful in phobic anxiety disorders. Specific serotonin reuptake inhibitors (SSRIs), e.g. **citalopram**, may be effective in panic disorder (Chapter 28).

Drugs acting at serotonergic (5HT) receptors

Serotonergic (5HT) cell bodies are located in the raphe nuclei of the midbrain and project to many areas of the brain, including those thought to be important in anxiety (hippocampus, amygdala, frontal cortex). In rats, lesions of the raphe nuclei produce anxiolytic effects, and BDZs microinjected into the dorsal raphe nucleus reduce the rate of neuronal firing and produce an anxiolytic effect. These experiments suggested that 5HT antagonists might be useful anxiolytic drugs. **Buspirone**, a $5HT_{1A}$ partial agonist, has anxiolytic actions in humans, perhaps by acting as an antagonist at postsynaptic $5HT_{1A}$ sites in the hippocampus (where there is little receptor reserve). Buspirone is not sedative and does not cause dependence. Unfortunately, it is only anxiolytic after 2 weeks of administration, and the indications for buspirone are unclear.

Chloral hydrate is converted in the body to trichloroethanol, which is an effective hypnotic. It may cause tolerance and dependence. Chloral hydrate can cause gastric irritation, but it is less likely to accumulate than the BDZs. It is little used nowadays.

Clomethiazole has no advantage over short-acting BDZs, except in the elderly, where it may cause less hangover. It is given by intravenous infusion in cases of acute alcohol withdrawal and in status epilepticus. Clomethiazole causes dependence and should be used only for a limited period.

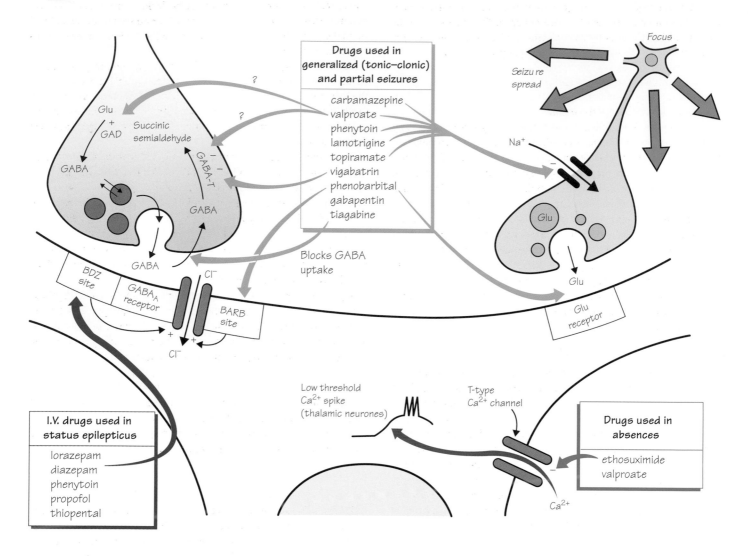

Epilepsy is a chronic disease in which seizures result from the abnormal discharge of cerebral neurones. The seizures are classified empirically.

Partial (focal) seizures begin at a specific locus (upper right figure) in the brain and may be limited to clonic jerking of an extremity. However, the discharge may spread (➡) and become generalized (**secondarily generalized seizure**). **Primarily generalized seizures** are those in which there is no evidence of localized onset, both cerebral hemispheres being involved from the onset. They include **tonic–clonic** attacks (*grand mal* – periods of tonic rigidity followed later by massive jerking of the body) and **absences** (*petit mal* – changes in consciousness usually lasting less than 10 s).

Generalized tonic–clonic seizures and partial seizures are treated mainly with oral **carbamazepine** (top middle), **valproate**, **lamotrigine** or **topiramate**. These drugs are of similar effectiveness, and a single drug will control the fits in 70–80% of patients with tonic–clonic seizures, but in only 30–40% of patients with partial seizures. In these poorly controlled patients, combinations of the above drugs or the addition of second-line drugs, e.g., **levetiracetam**, **clobazam** or

gabapentin may reduce the incidence of seizures, but only about 7% of these refractory patients become totally seizure free.

Absence seizures are treated with **ethosuximide** (bottom right) or **valproate**. Lamotrigine is also effective. Absence epilepsy only occasionally continues into adult life, but at least 10% of children will later develop tonic–clonic seizures.

Status epilepticus is defined as continuous seizures lasting at least 30 min or a state in which fits follow each other without consciousness being fully regained. Urgent treatment with **intravenous agents** (bottom left) is necessary to stop the fits, which, if unchecked, result in exhaustion and cerebral damage. **Lorazepam** or diazepam is used initially followed by **phenytoin** if necessary. If the fits are not controlled, the patient is anaesthetized with **propofol** or **thiopental**.

Antiepileptic drugs control seizures by mechanisms that usually involve either the enhancement of γ-aminobutyric acid (GABA)-mediated inhibition (left of figure) or a reduction of Na^+ fluxes (right of figure). Ethosuximide and valproate may inhibit a spike-generating Ca^{2+} current in thalamic neurones (bottom right).

Causes of epilepsy

The aetiology is unknown in 60–70% of cases, but heredity is an important factor. Damage to the brain (e.g. tumours, asphyxia, infections or head injury) may subsequently cause epilepsy. Convulsions may be precipitated in epileptics by several groups of drugs, including *phenothiazines*, *tricyclic antidepressants* and many *antihistamines*.

Mechanisms of action of anticonvulsants

Inhibition of sodium channels

Carbamazepine, **lamotrigine**, **valproate**, **phenytoin** and probably **topiramate** act by producing a use-dependent block of neuronal Na$^+$ channels. Their anticonvulsant action is a result of their ability to *prevent high-frequency repetitive activity*. The drugs bind preferentially to inactivated (closed) Na$^+$ channels, stabilizing them in the inactivated state and preventing them from returning to the resting (closed) state, which they must re-enter before they can again open (see Chapter 5). High-frequency repetitive depolarization increases the proportion of Na$^+$ channels in the inactivated state and, because these are susceptible to blockade by the antiepileptics, the Na$^+$ current is progressively reduced until it is eventually insufficient to evoke an action potential. Neuronal transmission at normal frequencies is relatively unaffected because a much smaller proportion of the Na$^+$ channels are in the inactivated state.

Enhancement of GABA action

Vigabatrin is an irreversible inhibitor of GABA-transaminase, which increases brain GABA levels and central GABA release. **Tiagabine** inhibits the reuptake of GABA, and by increasing the amount of GABA in the synaptic cleft, increases central inhibition. The benzodiazepines (e.g. **clobazam**, **clonazepam**) and **phenobarbital** also increase central inhibition, by enhancing the action of synaptically released GABA at the GABA$_A$ receptor–Cl$^-$ channel complex (Chapter 24). Phenobarbital may also reduce the effects of glutamate at excitatory synapses. **Valproate** also seems to increase GABAergic central inhibition by mechanisms that may involve stimulation of glutamic acid decarboxylase activity and/or inhibition of GABA-T.

Inhibition of calcium channels

Absence seizures involve oscillatory neuronal activity between the thalamus and cerebral cortex. This oscillation involves (T-type) Ca^{2+} channels in the thalamic neurones, which produce low threshold spikes and allow the cells to fire in bursts. Drugs that control absences (**ethosuximide**, **valproate** and **lamotrigine**) reduce this Ca^{2+} current, dampening the thalamocortical oscillations that are critical in the generation of absence seizures.

Drugs used in partial and generalized tonic–clonic (grand mal) seizures

Treatment with a single drug is preferred because this reduces adverse effects and drug interactions. Furthermore, most patients obtain no extra benefit from multiple drug regimens. **Carbamazepine** and **valproate** are the first-line drugs in epilepsy because they cause relatively few adverse effects and seem to have least detrimental effects on cognitive function and behaviour. Some anticonvulsants, especially phenytoin, phenobarbital and carbamazepine, are potent *liver enzyme inducers* and stimulate the metabolism of many drugs, e.g. oral contraceptives, warfarin, theophylline.

Carbamazepine is metabolized in the liver to carbamazepine-10, 11-epoxide, an active metabolite that partly contributes to both its anticonvulsant action and neurotoxicity. Mild neurotoxic effects are common (nausea, dizziness, drowsiness, blurred vision and ataxia) and often determine the limit of dosage. Agranulocytosis is a rarer idiosyncratic reaction to carbamazepine.

Phenytoin is hydroxylated in the liver by a saturable enzyme system. Measurement of serum drug levels is extremely valuable because, once the metabolizing enzymes are saturated, a small increase in dose may produce toxic blood levels of the drug. *Adverse effects* include ataxia, nystagmus gum hypertrophy, acne, greasy skin, coarsening of the facial features and hirsutism.

Topiramate blocks sodium channels in cultured neurones. It also enhances the effects of GABA and blocks α-amino-3-hydroxy-5-methyl-4-isoxazolepropionic acid (AMPA) receptors. Adverse effects include nausea, abdominal pain and anorexia. Topiramate has been associated with acute myopia and secondary closed-angle glaucoma.

Phenobarbital is probably as effective as carbamazepine and phenytoin in the treatment of tonic–clonic and partial seizures, but it is much more sedative. Tolerance occurs with prolonged use and sudden withdrawal may precipitate status epilepticus.

Vigabatrin, **gabapentin**, **levetiracetam**, **pregabalin** and **tiagabine** are used as 'add-on' drugs in patients in whom epilepsy is not satisfactorily controlled by other antiepileptics. Gabapentin (and carbamazepine) are also used to relieve *shooting and stabbing neuropathic pain* that responds poorly to conventional analgesics.

Drugs used to treat absences (petit mal)

Ethosuximide is only effective in the treatment of absences and myoclonic seizures (brief jerky movements without loss of consciousness). It is widely used as an anti-absence drug because it has relatively mild adverse effects (e.g. nausea, vomiting).

Drugs effective in tonic–clonic (grand mal) and absence (petit mal) seizures

Valproate. The advantages of valproate are its relative lack of sedative effects, its wide spectrum of activity and the mild nature of most of its adverse effects (nausea, weight gain, bleeding tendencies and transient hair loss). The main disadvantage is that occasional idiosyncratic responses cause *severe or fatal hepatic toxicity*.

Lamotrigine is used alone or in combination with other agents. Adverse effects include blurred vision, dizziness and drowsiness. Serious skin reactions may occur, especially in children. These include Stevens–Johnson syndrome and toxic epidermal necrolysis.

Benzodiazepines. **Clonazepam** is a potent anticonvulsant but is very sedative and tolerance occurs with prolonged oral administration.

Drug withdrawal

Abrupt withdrawal of antiepileptic drugs can cause rebound seizures. It is difficult to know when to withdraw antiepileptics but, if a patient has been seizure-free for 3 or 4 years, gradual withdrawal may be tried.

Pregnancy

Anticonvulsant therapy in pregnancy requires care because of the teratogenic potential of many of these drugs, especially valproate and phenytoin. Also there is concern that *in utero* exposure to valproate may damage neuropsychological development even in the absence of physical malformation.

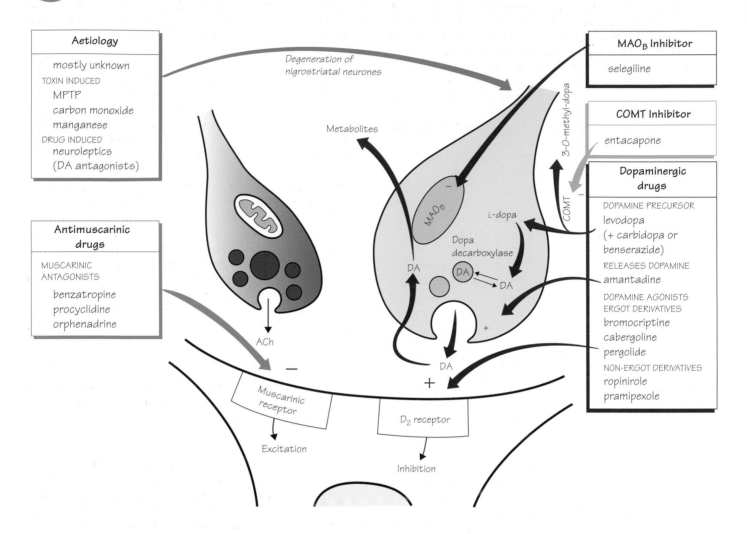

Parkinson's disease is a disease of the basal ganglia and is characterized by a poverty of movement, rigidity and tremor. It is progressive and leads to increasing disability unless effective treatment is given.

In the early 1960s, analysis of brains of patients dying with Parkinson's disease revealed greatly decreased levels of **dopamine** (DA) in the **basal ganglia** (caudate nucleus, putamen, globus pallidus). Parkinson's disease thus became the first disease to be associated with a specific transmitter abnormality in the brain. The main pathology in Parkinson's disease is extensive degeneration of the dopaminergic **nigrostriatal tract** (⟶), but the cause of the degeneration is usually unknown (top left). The cell bodies of this tract are localized in the substantia nigra in the midbrain, and it seems that frank symptoms of Parkinson's disease appear only when more than 80% of these neurones have degenerated. About one-third of patients with Parkinson's disease eventually develop dementia.

Replacement therapy with dopamine itself is not possible in Parkinson's disease because dopamine does not pass the blood–brain barrier. However, its precursor, **levodopa** (L-dopa), does penetrate the brain, where it is decarboxylated to dopamine (right figure). When orally administered, levodopa is largely metabolized outside the brain, and so it is given with a selective *extracerebral decarboxylase inhibitor*

(**carbidopa** or **benserazide**). This greatly decreases the effective dose by reducing peripheral metabolites and reduces peripheral adverse effects (*nausea, postural hypotension*). Levodopa, together with a peripheral decarboxylase inhibitor, is the mainstay of treatment. Other dopaminergic drugs used in Parkinson's disease (bottom right) are directly acting **dopamine agonists** and **amantadine**, which causes dopamine release. Some of the peripheral side-effects of dopaminergic drugs can be reduced with **domperidone**, a dopamine antagonist that does not penetrate the brain. Inhibition of monoamine oxidase B (MAO$_B$) with **selegiline** (top right) potentiates the actions of levodopa. **Entacapone** inhibits catechol-*O*-methyltransferase (COMT) and prevents the peripheral conversion of levodopa to (inactive) 3-*O*-methyldopa. It increases the plasma half-life of levodopa and increases its action.

As the nigrostriatal neurones progressively degenerate in Parkinson's disease, the release of (inhibitory) dopamine declines and the excitatory cholinergic interneurones in the striatum become relatively 'overactive' (left, ▭). This simple idea provides the rationale for treatment with **antimuscarinic agents** (bottom left). They are most useful in controlling the tremor that is usually the presenting feature in Parkinson's disease. Withdrawal of antimuscarinic drugs may worsen symptoms.

Aetiology

The cause of Parkinson's disease is unknown and no endogenous or environmental neurotoxin has been discovered. However, the possibility that such a chemical exists has been suggested dramatically by the discovery in Californian drug addicts (who were trying to make pethidine) that 1-methyl-4-phenyl-1,2,3,6-tetrahydropyridine (MPTP) causes degeneration of the nigrostriatal tract and Parkinson's disease. MPTP acts indirectly via a metabolite, 1-methyl-4-phenylpyridine (MPP^+), which is formed by the action of MAO_B. It is not certain how MPP^+ kills dopaminergic nerve cells, but free radicals generated during its formation by MAO_B may poison mitochondria and/or damage the cell membrane by peroxidation.

Antipsychotic drugs (Chapter 27) block dopamine receptors and often produce a Parkinson's disease-like syndrome.

Dopaminergic drugs

Levodopa with a selective extracerebral decarboxylase inhibitor is the most effective treatment for most patients with Parkinson's disease.

Mechanism of action

Levodopa is the immediate precursor of dopamine and is able to penetrate the brain, where it is converted to dopamine. The site of this decarboxylation in the parkinsonian brain is uncertain, but as dopa decarboxylase is not rate limiting, there may be sufficient enzyme in the remaining dopaminergic nerve terminals. Another possibility is that the conversion occurs in noradrenergic or serotonergic terminals, because the decarboxylase activity in these neurones is not specific. In any event, the release of dopamine replaced in the brain by levodopa therapy must be very abnormal, and it is remarkable that most patients with Parkinson's disease benefit, often dramatically, from its administration.

Adverse effects

Adverse effects are frequent, and mainly result from widespread stimulation of dopamine receptors. *Nausea* and *vomiting* are caused by stimulation of the chemoreceptor trigger zone (CTZ) in the area postrema, which lies outside the blood–brain barrier. This can be reduced by the peripherally acting dopamine antagonist domperidone. Psychiatric side-effects are the most common limiting factor in levodopa treatment and include vivid dreams, hallucinations, psychotic states and confusion. These effects are probably caused by stimulation of mesolimbic or mesocortical dopamine receptors (remember overactivity in these systems is associated with schizophrenia). Postural hypotension is common, but often asymptomatic. *Dyskinesias* are an important adverse effect that, in the early stages of Parkinson's disease, usually reflect overtreatment and respond to simple dose reduction (or fractionation).

Problems with long-term treatment

After 5 years' treatment, about 50% of patients will have lost ground. In some there is a gradual recurrence of parkinsonian akinesia. A second form of deterioration is the shortening of duration of action of each dose of levodopa ('*end-of-dose deterioration*'). Various dyskinesias may appear and, with time, many patients start to experience increasingly severe and rapid oscillations in mobility and dyskinesias – the '*on–off effect*'. These fluctuations in response are related to the peaks and troughs of plasma levodopa levels.

Dopamine agonists

These include ergot derivatives, e.g. **bromocriptine**, and newer non-ergot drugs, e.g. **ropinirole**. The ergot derivatives may cause fibrotic changes leading to restrictive valvular heart disease. This was thought to be rare, but in one study, pergolide was associated with valvular effects in 30% of patients. Dopamine agonists have no advantage over levodopa and the adverse effects are similar (nausea, psychiatric symptoms, postural hypotension). Most patients benefit initially from levodopa therapy, but views differ as to whether the later development of dyskinesias and unpredictable 'on–off' effects are caused by the cumulative dose of levodopa or just reflect progression of the disease. For this reason, younger patients in particular are often given a dopamine agonist as initial therapy (sometimes together with selegiline). This strategy may slow the development of dyskinesias, but only about 50% of patients show any beneficial response to monotherapy with dopamine agonists.

When patients on levodopa therapy start to show deterioration, dopamine agonists are often added to try to reduce the 'off' periods. In late disease, it seems that progressive neuronal degeneration reduces the capacity of the striatum to buffer fluctuating levodopa levels, because continuous dopaminergic stimulation produced by the intravenous infusion of levodopa, or subcutaneous infusion of apomorphine, controls the dyskinesias. Unfortunately, this form of treatment is not generally practical, but a simpler strategy of combining oral levodopa with single injections of apomorphine given during the 'off' periods helps many advanced fluctuating parkinsonian patients to have a more stable day.

Drugs causing dopamine release

Amantadine has muscarinic blocking actions and probably increases dopamine release. It has modest antiparkinsonian effects in a few patients, but tolerance soon occurs.

MAO_B and COMT inhibitors

Selegiline selectively inhibits MAO_B present in the brain, for which dopamine, but neither norepinephrine nor serotonin, is a substrate. It reduces the metabolism of dopamine in the brain and potentiates the actions of levodopa, the dose of which can be reduced by up to one-third. Because selegiline protects animals from the effects of MPTP, it was hoped that the drug might slow the progression of Parkinson's disease in patients. However, it seems that selegiline may actually increase mortality. Selegiline has a mild antiparkinsonian action when used alone and can delay the need for levodopa. It is also used in late disease as an adjunct to levodopa.

Entacapone inhibits COMT. It slows the elimination of levodopa and prolongs the duration of a single dose. It has no antiparkinsonian action alone, but initial studies suggest that it augments the action of levodopa and reduces the 'off' time in late disease.

Antimuscarinics

Muscarinic antagonists produce a modest improvement in the early stages of Parkinson's disease, but the akinesia that is responsible for most of the functional disability responds least well. Furthermore, adverse effects are common and include dry mouth, urinary retention and constipation. More seriously, antimuscarinics can affect memory and concentration and precipitate an organic confusional state with visual hallucinations, especially in elderly or dementing patients. The main use of these drugs is in the treatment of drug-induced parkinsonism (Chapter 27).

27 Antipsychotic drugs (neuroleptics)

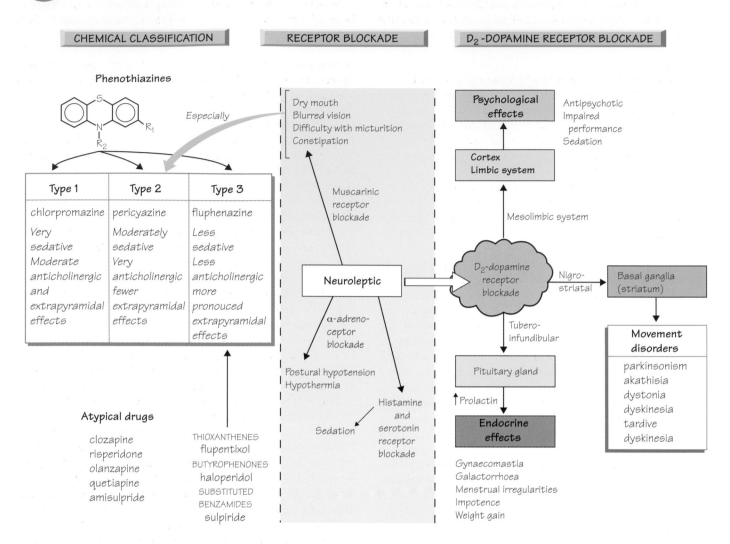

Schizophrenia is a syndrome characterized by specific psychological manifestations. These include auditory hallucinations, delusions, thought disorders and behavioural disturbances. It is thought that schizophrenia is caused by developmental abnormalities involving the medial temporal lobe (parahippocampal gyrus, hippocampus and amygdala), temporal and frontal lobe cortex. Schizophrenia can be a genetically determined illness, but there is also evidence implicating intrauterine events and obstetric complications. Neuroleptic drugs control many of the symptoms of schizophrenia. They have most effect on the positive symptoms, such as hallucinations and delusion. Negative symptoms, such as social withdrawal and emotional apathy, are less affected by neuroleptic drugs. About 30% of patients show only limited improvement, and 7% show no improvement even with prolonged treatment. The neuroleptics are all **antagonists at dopamine receptors**, suggesting that schizophrenia is associated with increased activity in the dopaminergic *mesolimbic* and/or *mesocortical pathway* (top right). In agreement with this idea, amfetamine (which causes dopamine release) can produce a psychotic state in normal subjects. Experiments using single photon emission computed tomography (SPECT) have shown that, in schizophrenics, there is a greater occupancy of D_2-receptors, implying greater dopaminergic stimulation.

Neuroleptic drugs require several weeks to control the symptoms of schizophrenia, and most patients will require maintenance treatment for many years. Relapses are common even in drug-maintained patients, and more than two-thirds of patients relapse within 1 year if they stop drug treatment. Unfortunately, neuroleptics also block dopamine receptors in the basal ganglia, and this frequently results in distressing and disabling **movement disorders** (extrapyramidal effects, right). These include parkinsonism, acute dystonic reactions (which may require treatment with antimuscarinic drugs), akathisia (motor restlessness) and tardive dyskinesia (orofacial and trunk movements), which may be irreversible. It is not known what causes tardive dyskinesia but, because it may be made worse by removing the drug, it has been suggested that the striatal dopamine receptors become supersensitive. Some 'atypical' drugs (bottom left) are free or relatively free of extrapyramidal side-effects at low doses.

In the pituitary gland, dopamine acting on D_2-dopamine receptors inhibits prolactin release. This effect is blocked by neuroleptics, and the resulting increase in prolactin release often causes **endocrine side-effects** (bottom right).

Many neuroleptics have muscarinic receptor and α-adrenoceptor blocking actions and cause **autonomic side-effects** (middle shaded yellow), including postural hypotension, dry mouth and constipation. The potency of individual drugs in blocking autonomic receptors, and therefore their predominant peripheral side-effects, depends on the **chemical class** to which they belong (left). Up to 1% of patients using antipsychotics develop **neuroleptic malignant syndrome**, a rare but potentially fatal idiosyncratic reaction that involves hyperthermia and muscle rigidity. Antipsychotic therapy is stopped immediately but there is no proven effective treatment. Cooling, dopaminergic agonists (e.g. bromocriptine) and dantrolene may be helpful, but the syndrome is fatal in 12–15% of cases.

Dopamine receptors

Dopamine receptors were originally subdivided into two types (D_1 and D_2). Currently, there are five cloned dopamine receptors that fall into these two classes. The D_1-like receptors include D_1 and D_5, while the D_2-like receptors include D_2, D_3 and D_4. The dopamine receptors all display the seven transmembrane-spanning domains characteristic of G-protein-linked receptors and are linked to adenylyl cyclase stimulation (D_1) or inhibition (D_2).

D_1-like dopamine receptors (subtypes D_1, D_5) are involved mainly in postsynaptic inhibition. Most neuroleptic drugs block D_1 receptors, but this action does not correlate with their antipsychotic activity. In particular, the *butyrophenones* are potent neuroleptics, but are weak D_1-receptor antagonists.

D_2-like dopamine receptors (subtypes D_2, D_3, D_4) are involved in presynaptic and postsynaptic inhibition. The D_2 receptor is the predominant subtype in the brain and is involved in most of the known functions of dopamine. D_2 receptors occur in the limbic system, which is concerned with mood and emotional stability, and in the basal ganglia, where they are involved in the control of movement. There are far fewer D_3 and D_4 receptors in the brain and they are located mainly in the limbic areas, where they may be involved in cognition and emotion.

Mechanism of action of neuroleptics

The affinity of neuroleptic drugs for the D_2 receptor correlates closely with their antipsychotic potency, and the blockade of D_2 receptors in the forebrain is believed to underlie their therapeutic actions. Unfortunately, blockade of D_2 receptors in the basal ganglia usually results in movement disorders. Some neuroleptics, in addition to blocking D_2 receptors, are also antagonists at $5HT_2$ receptors, and it is thought by some that this may somehow reduce the movement disorders caused by D_2 antagonism.

Chemical classification

Drugs with a wide variety of structures have antipsychotic activity, but they all have in common the ability to block dopamine receptors.

Phenothiazines

Phenothiazines are subdivided according to the type of side-chain attached to the N-atom of the phenothiazine ring.

Type 1: Propylamine side-chain

Phenothiazines with an aliphatic side-chain have relatively low potency and produce nearly all of the side-effects shown in the figure. **Chlorpromazine** was the first phenothiazine used in schizophrenia and is widely used, although it produces more adverse effects than newer drugs. It is very sedative and is particularly useful in treating violent patients. Adverse effects include sensitivity reactions, such as agranulocytosis, haemolytic anaemia, rashes, cholestatic jaundice and photosensitization.

Type 2: Piperidine side-chain

The main drug in this group was **thioridazine**. It was the first drug to be relatively rarely associated with movement disorders, perhaps because of its potent antimuscarinic effects. Unfortunately, thioridazine was associated with ventricular arrhythmias, conduction block and sudden death and has been withdrawn.

Type 3: Piperazine side-chain

Drugs in this group include **fluphenazine**, **perphenazine** and **trifluoperazine**. They are less sedative and less anticholinergic than chlorpromazine, but are particularly likely to cause movement disorders, especially in the elderly.

Other chemical classes

Butyrophenones. Haloperidol has little anticholinergic action and is less sedative and hypotensive than chlorpromazine. However, there is a high incidence of movement disorders.

Atypical drugs are so called because they are associated with a lower incidence of movement disorders and are better tolerated than other antipsychotics.

Clozapine is regarded by some as the only truly atypical neuroleptic because it is sometimes effective in patients refractory to other neuroleptic drugs. The drug is restricted to this group of refractory patients because it causes neutropenia in about 3%, and potentially fatal agranulocytosis in about 1% of patients (blood samples are required regularly to monitor white cells). Clozapine may be atypical because, at clinically effective doses, it blocks D_4 receptors (present mainly in limbic areas) with relatively little effect on striatal D_2 receptors. However, a specific D_4 antagonist was completely devoid of antipsychotic activity. Clozapine blocks many other receptors (centre figure) including muscarinic and $5HT_2$ receptors. Because antimuscarinic drugs abort neuroleptic-induced movement disorders, it is possible that blockade of muscarinic receptors accounts for the atypical action of clozapine, but **thioridazine**, which also has a high affinity for muscarinic receptors, may cause extrapyramidal effects at higher doses. Another suggestion is that the atypical action of clozapine is because of its potent block of $5HT_2$ receptors. This idea is supported by clinical trials in which ritanserin (a $5HT_2$ antagonist) apparently reduced the movement disorders caused by classic neuroleptics.

Risperidone is a newer drug that is non-sedative and lacks anticholinergic and α-blocking actions. It blocks $5HT_2$ receptors, but is a more potent antagonist than clozapine at D_2 receptors. At low doses, it does not cause extrapyramidal effects, but this advantage is lost with higher doses.

Sulpiride is a very specific D_2-blocker that is widely used because it has a low liability for extrapyramidal effects and, although quite sedating, can be well tolerated. It has been suggested that sulpiride has a higher affinity for mesolimbic D_2 receptors than striatal D_2 receptors.

Depot preparations

Schizophrenic patients are now often being 'returned to the community'. This has led to an increased use of long-acting depot injections for maintenance therapy. Oily injections of the decanoate derivatives of **flupenthixol**, **haloperidol**, **risperidone** and **fluphenazine** may be given by deep intramuscular injection at intervals of 1–4 weeks, but these preparations increase the incidence of movement disorders.

28 Drugs used in affective disorders: antidepressants

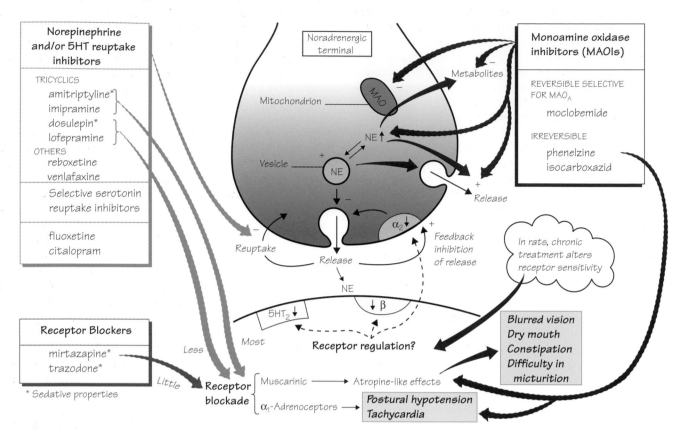

Affective disorders are characterized by a disturbance of mood associated with alterations in behaviour, energy, appetite, sleep and weight. The extremes range from intense excitement and elation (**mania**) to severe **depressive states**. In depression, which is much more common than mania, a person becomes persistently sad and unhappy. Depression is common and, although it can cause people to kill themselves, in general the prognosis is good.

Most of the drugs used in the treatment of depression inhibit the reuptake of norepinephrine (NE) and/or serotonin (5HT) (top left). The **tricyclics** are older drugs with proven efficacy, but are often sedative and have autonomic side-effects (▢) that may limit their use. The tricyclics are the most dangerous in overdosage, mainly because of cardiotoxicity, but convulsions are common. **Selective serotonin reuptake inhibitors** (SSRIs) have a wide margin of safety and a different spectrum of side-effects (mainly gastrointestinal). **Monoamine oxidase inhibitors** (MAOIs, top right) are used less often than other antidepressants because of dangerous interactions with some foods and drugs. A few antidepressants are **receptor blockers** and do not inhibit MAO or monoamine uptake (bottom left).

All antidepressants may provoke seizures, and no particular drug is safe for the depressed epileptic patient. A striking characteristic of antidepressant treatment with drugs is that the benefit does not become apparent for 2–3 weeks. The reason for this is unknown, but may be related to gradual changes in the sensitivity of central 5HT and/or adrenoceptors (▢). About 70% of patients respond satisfactorily to treatment with antidepressant drugs. If after trying single drugs from different classes no response is obtained, a second augmenting drug can be added, usually **lithium**. Other possibilities include tryptophan (the precursor of 5HT) and electroconvulsive therapy (ECT). Following a response, antidepressant drugs should be continued for 4–6 months because this reduces the incidence of relapse. Abrupt withdrawal of antidepressant drugs, especially MAOIs, may cause nausea, vomiting, panic, anxiety and motor restlessness.

The cause of depression and the mechanism of action of antidepressants are unknown. The **monoamine theory** was based on the idea that depression resulted from a decrease in the activity of central noradrenergic and/or serotonergic systems. There are problems with this theory, but it has not been replaced with a better one. More recently, interest has focused on the **mechanism of action** of antidepressants.

In *mania* and in *bipolar affective disorders* (where mania alternates with depression), **lithium** has a mood-stabilizing action. Lithium salts have a low therapeutic/toxic ratio and adverse effects are common. **Carbamazepine, gabapentin** and **valproate** also have mood-stabilizing properties and can be used in cases of non-response or intolerance to lithium.

Monoamine theory of depression

Reserpine, which depletes the brain of norepinephrine and serotonin, often causes depression. In contrast, the *tricyclics* and related compounds block the reuptake of norepinephrine and/or serotonin, and the MAOIs increase the concentration of norepinephrine and/or serotonin in the brain. Both of these actions increase the amounts of norepinephrine and/or serotonin available in the synaptic cleft. These drug effects suggest that depression might be associated with a decrease in brain norepinephrine and/or serotonin function, but it has proved difficult to find the expected defects in central noradrenergic and serotonergic systems in depressed patients. There are several problems with the monoamine theory of depression. In particular, it has been difficult to understand why the tricyclic drugs rapidly block norepinephrine/serotonin uptake but require weeks of administration to achieve an antidepressant effect. Recent evidence suggests that hippocampal neurodegeneration may be involved in depression.

Mechanism of action of antidepressants

The mechanisms involved in antidepressant action are poorly understood. It is thought that SSRIs cause an increase in extracellular serotonin that initially activates autoreceptors, an action that inhibits serotonin release and reduces extracellular serotonin to its previous level. However, with chronic treatment, the inhibitory autoreceptors desensitize and there is then a maintained increase in forebrain serotonin release that causes the therapeutic effects. Drugs that inhibit norepinephrine uptake probably act indirectly, either by stimulating the serotonergic neurones (which have an excitatory noradrenergic input) or by desensitizing inhibitory presynaptic α_2-receptors in the forebrain. In addition to α_2-adrenoceptors, the chronic administration of antidepressants to rodents also gradually decreases the sensitivity of central $5HT_2$ and β_1-adrenoceptors, but the significance of these changes is unknown. It is also unknown whether changes in receptor sensitivity are involved in the antidepressant action of drugs in humans, but chronic antidepressant treatment has been shown to lower the sensitivity of clonidine (an α_2-adrenoceptor agonist).

Drugs that inhibit amine uptake

The term '**tricyclic drug**' refers to compounds based on the dibenzazepine (e.g. **imipramine**) and dibenzocycloheptadiene (e.g. **amitriptyline**) ring structures. No individual tricyclic drug has superior antidepressant activity, and the choice of drug is determined by the most acceptable or desired side-effects. Thus, drugs with sedative actions such as **amitriptyline** and **dosulepin** are more suitable for agitated and anxious patients and, if given at bedtime, will also act as a hypnotic. The tricyclics resemble the phenothiazines in structure and have similar blocking actions at cholinergic *muscarinic receptors*, *α-adrenoceptors* and *histamine receptors*. These actions frequently cause dry mouth, blurred vision, constipation, urinary retention, tachycardia and postural hypotension. In overdosage, the anticholinergic activity and quinidine-like action of the tricyclics on the heart may cause arrhythmias and sudden death. *They are contraindicated in heart disease.*

The SSRIs do not have the troublesome autonomic side-effects or appetite-stimulating effects of the tricyclics, but do have different ones, the most common being nausea, vomiting, diarrhoea and constipation. They may also cause sexual dysfunction. The SSRIs are now generally accepted as first-line drugs, especially in patients with cardiovascular disease, those in whom any sedation must be avoided, or for those who cannot tolerate the anticholinergic effects of the tricyclics. SSRIs should not be given to patients under 18 years of age because they may increase the risk of suicidal behaviour. **Venlafaxine** inhibits the reuptake of both 5HT and (at higher doses) norepinephrine, and may have greater efficacy than other antidepressants. Its adverse effects generally resemble those of the SSRIs.

Receptor blockers

These drugs have little or no effect on amine uptake. They generally cause fewer autonomic side-effects and, because they are less cardiotoxic, they are less dangerous in overdosage. **Mirtazapine** and **trazodone** are sedative antidepressants. Mirtazapine has α_2-adrenoceptor blocking activity and, by blocking inhibitory α_2-autoreceptors on central noradrenergic nerve endings, it may increase the amount of norepinephrine in the synaptic cleft. Trazodone blocks $5HT_2$ and H_1-histamine receptors it also increases 5HT and noradrenaline release.

Monoamine oxidase inhibitors

The older MAOIs (e.g. **phenelzine**) are irreversible non-selective inhibitors of monoamine oxidase. They are rarely used now because of their adverse effects (postural hypotension, dizziness, anticholinergic effects and liver damage) and interactions with sympathomimetic amines (e.g. *ephedrine*, often present in cough mixtures and decongestive preparations) or foods containing *tyramine* (e.g. cheese, game, alcoholic drinks), which may result in severe hypertension. Ingested tyramine is normally metabolized by monoamine oxidase in the gut wall and liver, but when the enzyme is inhibited, tyramine reaches the circulation and causes the release of norepinephrine from sympathetic nerve endings (indirect sympathomimetic action). MAOIs are not specific and reduce the metabolism of barbiturates, opioid analgesics and alcohol. Pethidine is especially dangerous in patients taking MAOIs, causing – by an unknown mechanism – hyperpyrexia, hypotension and coma. **Moclobemide** is a reversible inhibitor that selectively inhibits monoamine oxidase A (cf. selegiline, Chapter 26). It is well tolerated, the main side-effects being dizziness, insomnia and nausea. Moclobemide interacts with the same drugs as other MAOIs but, because it is reversible, the effects of the interaction rapidly diminish when the drug is discontinued. Moclobemide is a second-line drug used in depression after tricyclics and SSRIs.

Lithium

Lithium is used for prophylaxis in *manic/depressive* illness. It is also used in treatment of acute mania but, because it may take several days for the antimanic effect to develop, an antipsychotic drug is usually preferred for acutely disturbed patients. Lithium is used as an **antidepressant** in combination with tricyclics in refractory patients.

Lithium is rapidly absorbed from the gut. The therapeutic and toxic doses are similar, and serum lithium concentrations must be measured regularly (therapeutic range: 0.4–1.0 mM). Adverse effects include nausea, vomiting, anorexia, diarrhoea, tremor of the hands, polydipsia and polyuria (a few patients develop nephrogenic diabetes insipidus), hypothyroidism and weight gain. Signs of *lithium toxicity* include drowsiness, ataxia and confusion and, at serum levels above 2–3 mM, life-threatening seizures and coma may occur.

Mechanism of action

This is unknown, but probably involves interactions with second messenger systems. In particular, lithium at concentrations of less than 1 mM blocks the phosphatidylinositol (PI) pathway at the point where inositol-1-phosphate is hydrolysed to inositol. This causes depletion of membrane phosphatidylinositol bisphosphate (PIP_2) (see Chapter 1) and may reduce the actions of transmitters acting at receptors that involve inositol-1,4,5-trisphosphate/diacylglycerol ($InsP_3$/DG) as their second messengers.

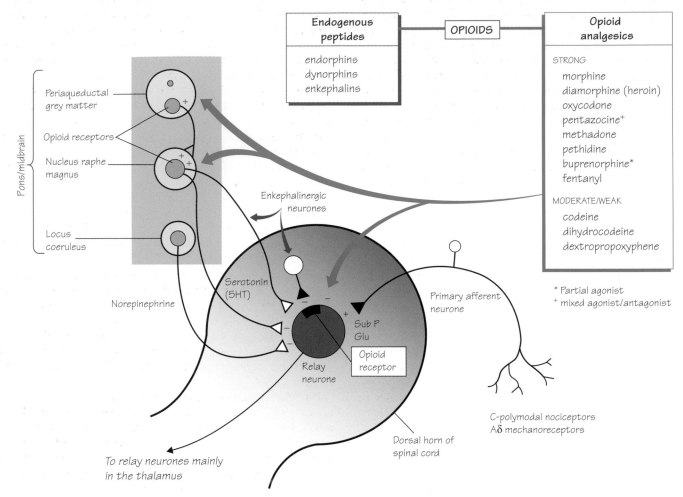

Endogenous peptides
endorphins
dynorphins
enkephalins

OPIOIDS

Opioid analgesics
STRONG
morphine
diamorphine (heroin)
oxycodone
pentazocine+
methadone
pethidine
buprenorphine*
fentanyl
MODERATE/WEAK
codeine
dihydrocodeine
dextropropoxyphene

* Partial agonist
\+ mixed agonist/antagonist

Damage to tissue causes the release of chemicals (e.g. bradykinin, prostaglandins, adenosine triphosphate [ATP], protons) that stimulate pain receptors (bottom, right) and initiate firing in primary afferent fibres that synapse in lamina I and II of the dorsal horn of the spinal cord. The relay neurones (⬤) in the dorsal horn transmit pain information to the sensory cortex via neurones in the thalamus. Little is known about the transmitter substances utilized in the ascending pain pathways, but primary afferent fibres release glutamate and peptides (e.g. substance P, calcitonin gene-related peptide) (lower figure, shaded). Neuropathic pain (shooting, burning sensation) is caused by damage to neurones in the pain pathway and often does not respond to opioids.

The activity of the dorsal horn relay neurones is modulated by several *inhibitory inputs*. These include local interneurones, which release **opioid peptides** (mainly dynorphin), and descending *enkephalinergic*, *noradrenergic* and *serotonergic* fibres, which originate in the brainstem (top left shaded orange) and are themselves activated by *opioid peptides*. Thus, opioid peptide release in both the brainstem and the spinal cord can *reduce* the activity of the dorsal horn relay neurones and can cause analgesia. The effects of opioid peptides are mediated by specific **opioid receptors**.

Opioid analgesics (right) are drugs that mimic endogenous opioid peptides by causing a prolonged activation of opioid receptors (usually μ-receptors). This produces analgesia, respiratory depression, euphoria

and sedation. Pain acts as an antagonist of respiratory depression, which may become a problem if the pain is removed, e.g. with a local anaesthetic. Opioids often cause nausea and vomiting, and antiemetics may be required. Effects on the nerve plexuses in the gut, which also possess opioid peptides and receptors, cause constipation, and laxatives are usually required (Chapter 13). Continuous treatment with opioid analgesics results in **tolerance** and **dependence** in addicts. However, in terminally ill patients, a steady increase in morphine dosage is not automatic and, where it does occur, is more likely to result from progressively increasing pain rather than tolerance. Similarly, in the clinical context, dependence is unimportant. *Unfortunately, overcaution in the use of opioid analgesics frequently results in unnecessarily poor pain control in patients.*

Some analgesics, such as **codeine** and **dihydrocodeine**, are less potent than morphine and cannot be given in equianalgesic doses because of the onset of adverse effects. As a result of this restriction in dosage, they are less likely, in practice, to produce respiratory depression and dependence. They are useful in controlling mild to moderate pain.

Naloxone is a specific antagonist at opioid receptors and reverses respiratory depression caused by morphine-like drugs. It also precipitates a withdrawal syndrome when dependence has occurred. Electro-acupuncture analgesia, transcutaneous nerve stimulation-induced analgesia and placebo effects can sometimes be partially blocked by naloxone, suggesting the involvement of the endogenous opioid peptides.

Opioids are defined as compounds with effects that are antagonized by naloxone. There are three families of **opioid peptides**, which are derived from large precursor molecules, encoded by separate genes. *Pro-opiomelanocortin* (POMC) gives rise to the opioid peptide β-endorphin and a number of other non-opioid peptides, including adrenocorticotrophic hormone (ACTH). *Proenkephalin* gives rise to leu-enkephalin and met-enkephalin. *Prodynorphin* gives rise to a number of opioid peptides, which contain leu-enkephalin at their amino terminal (e.g. dynorphin A). The peptides derived from each of these three precursor molecules have a distinct anatomical distribution in the central nervous system and have varying affinity for the different types of opioid receptors. The precise function of these opioid peptides in the brain and elsewhere is still unclear.

Opioid receptors are widely distributed throughout the central nervous system and have been classified into three main types. The μ-receptors are most highly concentrated in brain areas involved in nociception and are the receptors with which most opioid analgesics interact to produce analgesia (transgenic mice lacking μ-receptors are unresponsive to morphine). The δ- and κ-receptors display selectivity for the enkephalins and the dynorphins, respectively. Activation of κ-receptors also produces analgesia but, in contrast to μ-agonists (e.g. **morphine**), which cause euphoria, κ-agonists (e.g. **pentazocine**, **nalbuphine**) are associated with dysphoria. Some opioid analgesics (e.g. *pentazocine*) produce stimulant and psychotomimetic effects by acting on σ-receptors (phencyclidine, a psychotomimetic drug, binds to these receptors). Because these effects are not blocked by naloxone, σ-receptors are not opioid receptors. The opioid peptides have inhibitory actions on synapses in the central nervous system and gut. Opioid receptors are linked to G-proteins that open K^+ channels (causing hyperpolarization) and close Ca^{2+} channels (inhibiting transmitter release). Excitatory effects of opioids, e.g. in the pons/midbrain, are indirect, resulting from the inhibition of γ-aminobutyric acid (GABA) release.

Strong opioid analgesics

These are used particularly in the treatment of dull, poorly localized (visceral) pain. Somatic pain is sharply defined and may be relieved by a weak opioid analgesic or by a non-steroidal anti-inflammatory drug (NSAID, Chapter 32). **Parenteral morphine** is widely used to treat severe pain, whereas **oral morphine** is the drug of choice in terminal care.

Morphine and other opioid analgesics produce a range of central effects that include analgesia, euphoria, sedation, respiratory depression, depression of the vasomotor centre (causing postural hypotension), miosis because of IIIrd nerve nucleus stimulation (except pethidine, which has weak atropine-like activity), and nausea and vomiting caused by stimulation of the chemoreceptor trigger zone. They also cause cough suppression, but this is not correlated with their opioid activity. Peripheral effects, which include constipation, biliary spasm and constriction of the sphincter of Oddi, may occur. Morphine may cause histamine release with vasodilatation and itching. Morphine is metabolized in the liver by conjugation with glucuronic acid to form morphine-3-glucuronide, which is inactive, and morphine-6-glucuronide, which is a more potent analgesic than morphine itself, especially when given intrathecally.

Tolerance (i.e. decreased responsiveness) to many of the effects of opioid analgesics occurs with continuous administration. Miosis and constipation are effects to which little tolerance develops.

Both physical and psychological *dependence* on opioid analgesics gradually develops, and sudden termination of drug administration precipitates a withdrawal syndrome (Chapter 31).

Diamorphine (heroin, diacetylmorphine) is more lipid soluble than morphine and therefore has a more rapid onset of action when given by injection. The higher peak levels result in more sedation than that caused by morphine. Increasingly, small epidural doses of diamorphine are being used to control severe pain.

Fentanyl, **alfentanil** and **remifentanil** (Chapter 23) are potent, highly lipid-soluble, rapidly acting, μ-agonists. They are given intravenously to provide analgesia during maintenance anaesthesia. Low doses of fentanyl and alfentanil are short-acting due to rapid redistribution, but higher doses saturate the tissues and their actions are more prolonged. In contrast to fentanyl and alfentanil, which are metabolized by the liver, remifentanil is metabolized by tissue and blood esterases and has a constant $t_{1/2}$, even after prolonged infusion. Fentanyl may be given transdermally in patients with chronic stabilized pain, especially if oral opioids cause intractable nausea or vomiting. The fentanyl patches are not suitable for treating acute pain.

Methadone has a long duration of action and is less sedating than morphine. It is used orally for maintenance treatment of heroin or morphine addicts, in whom it prevents the 'buzz' of intravenous drugs (see also Chapter 31).

Pethidine has a rapid onset of action, but its short duration (3 h) makes it unsuitable for the control of prolonged pain. Pethidine is metabolized in the liver and, at high doses, a toxic metabolite (norpethidine) can accumulate and cause convulsions. Pethidine interacts seriously with monoamine oxidase inhibitors (MAOIs) (Chapter 28) causing delirium, hyperpyrexia and convulsions or respiratory depression.

Buprenorphine is a partial agonist at μ-receptors. It has a slow onset of action, but is an effective analgesic following sublingual administration. It has a much longer duration of action (6–8 h) than morphine, but may cause prolonged vomiting. Respiratory depression is rare but, if it occurs, is difficult to reverse with naloxone, because buprenorphine dissociates very slowly from the receptors.

Weak opioid analgesics

Weak opioid analgesics are used in 'mild-to-moderate' pain. They may cause dependence and are subject to abuse. However, they are less attractive to addicts because they do not give a good 'buzz'.

Codeine (methylmorphine) is well absorbed orally, but has a very low affinity for opioid receptors. About 10% of the drug is demethylated in the liver to morphine, which is responsible for the analgesic effects of codeine. Side-effects (constipation, vomiting, sedation) limit the possible dosage to levels that produce much less analgesia than morphine. Codeine is also used as an antitussive and antidiarrhoeal agent.

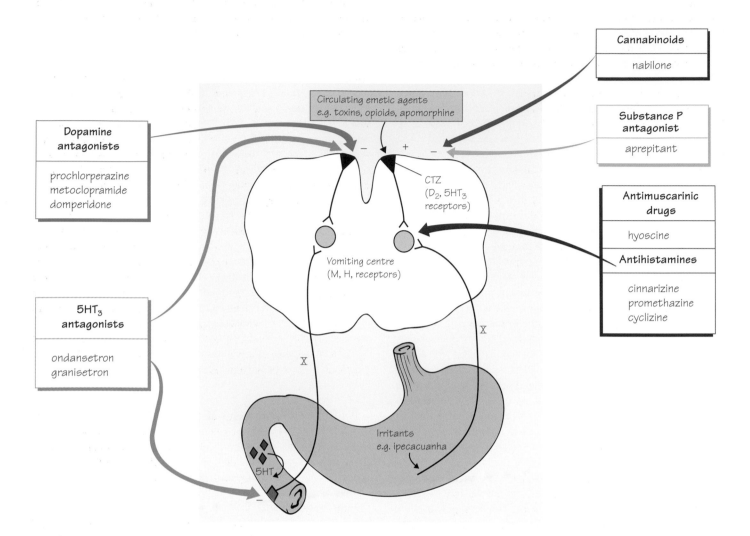

Nausea and vomiting have many causes, including drugs (e.g. cytotoxic agents, opioids, anaesthetics, digoxin), vestibular disease, provocative movement (e.g. seasickness), migraine and pregnancy. Vomiting is much easier to prevent than to stop once it has started. Therefore, if possible, antiemetics should be given well before the emetic stimulus is expected. Antiemetics should not be given before the diagnosis is known because identification of the underlying cause may be delayed.

Emesis is coordinated by the **vomiting centre** (⬤) in the medulla (upper figure). An important source of stimulation of the vomiting centre is the **chemoreceptor trigger zone** (CTZ, ▼) in the area postrema. Because the CTZ is not protected by the blood–brain barrier (it is part of the circumventricular system), it can be stimulated by circulating toxins or drugs (top). The CTZ possesses many dopamine (D_2) receptors, which explains why dopaminergic drugs used in the treatment of Parkinson's disease frequently cause nausea and vomiting. However, **dopamine receptor antagonists** are **antiemetics** (upper left) and are used to reduce nausea and vomiting associated with the administration of emetogenic drugs (e.g. many cytotoxic anticancer agents).

The CTZ also possesses $5HT_3$ receptors, and **$5HT_3$ antagonists** (e.g. ondansetron, left lower) are effective antiemetics. Because they have fewer unwanted actions, they are increasingly being used to prevent or reduce the nausea and vomiting associated with cancer chemotherapy and general anaesthesia. In some cases, it is uncertain how $5HT_3$ antagonists produce their antiemetic effects. There is a high concentration of $5HT_3$ receptors in the CTZ, but a peripheral action may also be important. Many cytotoxic drugs (and X-rays) cause the release of 5HT from enterochromaffin cells (◆) in the gut, and this activates $5HT_3$ receptors on vagal sensory fibres (◆) (lower figure). Stimulation of sensory fibres in the stomach by irritants (e.g. ipecacuanha, bacterial toxins) causes 'reflex' nausea and vomiting.

Dopamine antagonists and $5HT_3$ antagonists are ineffective in reducing the nausea and vomiting of **motion sickness**. **Antimuscarinic drugs** or **antihistamines** (right), which act directly on the vomiting centre, may be effective, although side-effects are common. Vertigo and vomiting associated with **vestibular disease** are treated with **antihistamines** (e.g. promethazine, cinnarizine), **phenothiazines** or **betahistine**.

Substance P given intravenously causes vomiting. Therefore, it was reasoned, antagonists of substance P might have an antiemetic action. This idea led to the introduction of **aprepitant**, a neurokinin-1 receptor antagonist.

The **vomiting centre** is in the lateral reticular formation of the medulla at the level of the olivary nuclei. It receives afferents from the following:

1 *Limbic cortex*. These afferents presumably account for the nausea associated with unpleasant odours and sights. Cortical afferents are also involved in the conditioned vomiting reflex that may occur when patients see or smell the cytotoxic drugs they are about to receive.

2 *CTZ*.

3 *Nucleus solitarius*. These afferents complete the arc for the gag reflex (i.e. the reflex caused by poking a finger in the mouth).

4 *Spinal cord* (spinoreticular fibres). These are involved in the nausea that accompanies physical injury.

5 *Vestibular system*. These are involved in the nausea and vomiting associated with vestibular disease and motion sickness.

The transmitters involved in the pathways concerned with emesis are not fully known. However, the CTZ is rich in D_2 dopamine and $5HT_3$ receptors. Cholinergic and histaminergic synapses are involved in transmission from the vestibular apparatus to the vomiting centre.

The vomiting centre projects to the vagus nerve and to the spinal motor neurones supplying the abdominal muscles. It is responsible for coordinating the complex events underlying emesis. Reverse peristalsis transfers the contents of the upper intestine into the stomach. The glottis closes, the breath is held, the oesophagus and gastric sphincter relax, and finally the abdominal muscles contract, ejecting the gastric contents.

Drug-induced vomiting

Cytotoxic drugs vary in their emetic potential, but some, e.g. cisplatin, cause severe vomiting in most patients. The emetic action of these drugs seems to involve the CTZ, and the dopamine antagonists are often effective antiemetics. **Prochlorperazine** is a phenothiazine that has been widely used as an antiemetic. It is less sedative than chlorpromazine, but may cause severe dystonic reactions (like all typical neuroleptics, Chapter 27). **Metoclopramide** is a D_2 antagonist, but also has a prokinetic action on the gut and increases the absorption of many drugs (Chapter 13). This can be an advantage, e.g. in migraine, where the absorption of analgesics is enhanced. Adverse effects are usually mild, but severe dystonic reactions may occur (more commonly in the young and in females). **Domperidone** is similar to metoclopramide, but does not cross the blood–brain barrier and rarely causes sedation or extrapyramidal effects. The $5HT_3$ antagonists, e.g. **ondansetron**, lack the adverse effects of dopamine antagonists, but may cause constipation or headaches. It has been shown in clinical trials that the severe vomiting caused by highly emetic cytotoxic drugs is controlled better by combinations of intravenous antiemetic drugs, e.g. **metoclopramide** and **dexamethasone**. A combination of **ondansetron** and **dexamethasone** will prevent cisplatin-induced emesis in most patients. It is not known why dexamethasone is antiemetic.

Aprepitant is a neurokinin-1 receptor antagonist that blocks the action of substance P in the CTZ. It is used as an adjunct to dexamethasone and a $5HT_3$ antagonist to prevent vomiting caused by cytotoxic chemotherapy. **Nabilone**, a synthetic cannabinoid, decreases vomiting caused by

agents that stimulate the CTZ. The mechanism of action is unknown but may involve opioid receptors because its antiemetic action is blocked by naloxone. It is used in cytotoxic chemotherapy when other antiemetics have been ineffective. Unwanted effects include drowsiness, dry mouth, hypotension and psychotic reactions.

Motion sickness

Motion sickness is very common and includes seasickness, airsickness, etc. It is characterized by pallor, cold sweating, nausea and vomiting. The symptoms and signs develop relatively gradually but eventually culminate in vomiting or retching, after which there is often a temporary lessening of malaise. Continued exposure to the provocative motion (e.g. of a ship) leads to increasing protective adaptation and, after 4 days, most people are symptom free. Motion sickness is believed to be a response to conflicting sensory information (i.e. signals from the eye and vestibular system do not agree). Little is known about the neural mechanisms involved in motion sickness, but it does not occur following labyrinthectomy or ablation of the vestibular cerebellum.

Procedures that reduce vestibular/visual conflict may help. For example, avoid head movements and, if on the deck of a ship, one should fixate on the horizon, but if enclosed in a cabin it is better to close one's eyes. **Hyoscine** is one of the most effective agents for reducing the incidence of motion sickness. It is a muscarinic receptor antagonist and frequently causes drowsiness, dry mouth and blurred vision. **Cinnarizine** is an antihistamine. It has an efficacy similar to that of hyoscine, but produces fewer side-effects. It must be taken 2 h before exposure to provocative stimulation.

Vestibular disease

The labyrinths generate a continuous input to the brainstem. Any pathological process that alters the balance of this *tonus* may cause dizziness (anything from lightness in the head to the inability to stand or walk). The major symptom is *vertigo*, which is a false sense of rotary movement, associated with sympathetic overactivity, nausea and vomiting.

Acute labyrinthitis

Acute labyrinthitis often presents abruptly as vertigo with nausea and vomiting. It is frequently regarded as a viral or postviral syndrome. **Ménière's disease** results from increased pressure in the membranous labyrinth. Attacks of severe vertigo associated with nausea, vomiting, deafness and tinnitus occur several times, followed by long periods of remission. Between attacks, the deafness and tinnitus persist and gradually worsen. Antiemetics used in labyrinth disease include **antihistamines (cinnarizine, cyclizine)** and **phenothiazines (promethazine, prochlorperazine)**. **Betahistine** is a drug used specifically in Ménière's disease because it is supposed to act by reducing endolymphatic pressure.

Pregnancy

Antiemetics should only be used for intractable vomiting because of possible, but undefined, risk to the fetus. Limited evidence suggests that **promethazine** is safe.

31 Drug misuse and dependence

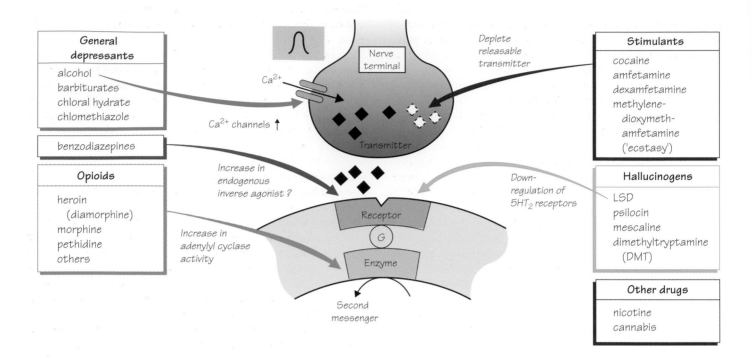

The relationship between society and drugs that act on the mind is one of an uneasy and changing coexistence. For example, there is much popular concern today about the illicit use of opioids, but in the nineteenth century, laudanum, an alcoholic solution of opium, was a popular and readily available home medication. Society now accepts only **alcohol** and **nicotine** (tobacco) as legal psychoactive drugs, although their misuse is responsible for considerable morbidity and mortality. Smoking is by far the most common form of drug dependency in the UK and causes 120 000 deaths each year in Britain; it is the biggest cause of avoidable premature death.

The term **drug misuse** is applied to any drug-taking that harms or threatens to harm the physical or mental health of an individual, or other individuals, or which is illegal. Thus, drug misuse includes *alcohol* and *nicotine* and the deleterious overprescription of medicines (e.g. **benzodiazepines**, **stimulants**), as well as the more obvious taking of illicit drugs.

Drug dependence is a term used when a person has a compulsion to take a drug in order to experience its psychic effects, and sometimes to avoid the discomfort of withdrawal symptoms.

The likelihood of drug misuse leading to dependence is determined by many factors, including the *type of drug*, the *route of administration*, the *pattern of drug-taking* and the *individual*. Rapid delivery systems (i.e. intravenous injection, smoking cocaine or heroin) increase the dependence potential. Intravenous injections have attendant dangers of infection (AIDS, hepatitis, septicaemia, etc.).

Drug dependence is often associated with **tolerance**, a phenomenon that may occur with chronic administration of a drug. It is characterized by the necessity to progressively increase the dose of the drug to produce its original effect. Tolerance may be caused, in part, by increased metabolism of the drug (pharmacokinetic tolerance), but is mainly caused by neuroadaptive changes in the brain.

The mechanisms underlying drug dependence and tolerance are poorly understood. In general, chronic drug administration induces homeostatic adaptive changes in the brain that operate so as to oppose the action of the drug. Withdrawal of the drug causes a rebound in central excitability. Thus, the withdrawal of depressants (e.g. alcohol, barbiturates) may result in convulsions, whereas the withdrawal of excitatory drugs (e.g. amfetamine) results in depression.

Many neuroadaptive changes in the brain have been described following chronic drug administration. They include an increase in Ca^{2+} channels (top left), depletion of transmitter (top right), receptor downregulation (middle right), changes in second messengers (bottom left) and the synthesis of an inverse agonist (middle left).

The brain circuits involved in drug dependence are not known. However, there is evidence from animal experiments that one important circuit is the dopaminergic pathway from the ventral tegmental area that projects to the nucleus accumbens and prefrontal cortex. By the use of microdialysis techniques, which can measure transmitter release from discrete brain areas, it has been shown that many drugs of dependence (e.g. stimulants, opioids, nicotine, alcohol) increase dopamine release in the nucleus accumbens and/or the frontal cortex. Some (e.g. amfetamine, cocaine) act on nerve terminals, whereas opioids increase dopamine release by inhibiting GABAergic input onto the dopaminergic neurones. Animals will self-administer cocaine and opioids into the nucleus accumbens, and the 'pleasure' this causes reinforces the self-administration. A similar reward system may be involved in human drug dependence. There is some evidence from experiments using positron emission tomography (PET) that drug abuse may be associated with a reduced concentration of D_2 dopamine receptors in the brain.

Central stimulants

Amfetamine-like drugs given orally decrease appetite, give a sense of increased energy and well-being, and enhance physical performance. They also have peripheral sympathomimetic effects (e.g. hypertension, tachycardia) and cause insomnia. Amfetamine-like drugs cause dopamine and norepinephrine release from nerve terminals, but their behavioural effects are caused mainly by dopamine release. **Cocaine** blocks the reuptake of dopamine into nerve terminals and has very similar effects to amfetamine. Cocaine hydrochloride is usually 'snorted' up the nose, but the free base ('crack'), which is more volatile, can be smoked, whereupon it is rapidly absorbed through the lungs and produces a sudden, brief, but overwhelming, sense of euphoria ('rush'). A similar 'rush' is produced by intravenous amfetamine, and addicts cannot distinguish between them. The *stimulants are highly addictive* and are psychotoxic. Repeated administration may produce a state resembling an acute attack of schizophrenia.

Methylene dioxymethamfetamine (**MDMA**, 'ecstasy') has mixed stimulant and hallucinogenic properties, the latter action perhaps resulting from 5-hydroxytryptamine (5HT) release. MDMA is widely abused as a 'recreational' drug, but has occasionally caused fatal acute hyperthermia. There is increasing evidence that long-term use of MDMA destroys 5HT nerve terminals and increases the risk of psychiatric disorders.

Opioids

Diamorphine (**heroin**) and other opioids have a high potential for misuse and dependence because of the intense sense of euphoria they produce when taken intravenously. Tolerance develops quickly in addicts, and abrupt withdrawal of opioids results in a craving to take the drug, together with a withdrawal syndrome characterized by yawning, sweating, gooseflesh, tremor, irritability, anorexia, nausea and vomiting. The substitution of oral long-acting drugs (**methadone** or **buprenorphine**) reduces the harm of heroin addiction (e.g. infection, criminality) and can be a stage to detoxification by gradually reducing the dose. The usual non-substitute method of detoxification is administration of **lofexidine**, a centrally acting α_2-agonist that can suppress some components of the withdrawal syndrome, especially the nausea, vomiting and diarrhoea. **Naltrexone**, an orally active opioid antagonist, prevents the euphoric action of opioids and is given daily to former addicts with the aim of preventing relapses.

The mechanisms underlying opioid dependence and tolerance are unknown. Chronic administration does not affect opioid receptors, but changes in second messengers may be important; e.g. in the *locus coeruleus*, μ-receptor activation inhibits adenylyl cyclase activity, but with chronic opioid administration the activity of the enzyme increases. Withdrawal of the inhibitory opioid then results in excessive cyclic adenosine monophosphate (cAMP) production, which may contribute to the rebound (increase) of neuronal excitability.

Hallucinogens (psychedelics)

Lysergic acid diethylamide (**LSD**) and related drugs induce dramatic states of altered perception, vivid and unusual sensory experiences and feelings of ecstasy. Occasionally, LSD produces unwanted effects, which include panic, frightening delusions and hallucinations. Usually the 'bad trip' fades away, but sometimes it returns later ('flashbacks').

Serotonergic systems may be important in the actions of LSD, which inhibits the firing of 5HT-containing neurones in the *raphe nuclei*, probably by stimulating $5HT_2$ inhibitory autoreceptors on these cells. Tolerance to LSD and related compounds occurs, and is associated with a downregulation of $5HT_2$ receptors. However, there is no withdrawal syndrome.

Cannabis (**marijuana**, **hashish**). The main active constituent of cannabis is Δ^9-tetrahydrocannabinol (THC). Cannabis has both hallucinogenic and depressant actions. It produces feelings of euphoria, relaxation and well-being. Cannabis is not dangerously addictive, but at least mild degrees of dependence may occur. Cannabis may cause acute psychotoxic effects that in some ways resemble an LSD 'bad trip'.

General depressants

Benzodiazepines are more readily available drugs, and **temazepam** is a popular drug of abuse, especially with opiate addicts, who use it to tide themselves over withdrawals.

Alcohol has effects that resemble those of general anaesthetics. It inhibits presynaptic Ca^{2+} entry (and hence transmitter release) and potentiates GABA-mediated inhibition. Considerable tolerance occurs to alcohol, but the mechanisms involved are poorly understood. Presynaptic Ca^{2+} channels may increase in number so that, when alcohol is withdrawn, transmitter release is abnormally high and this may contribute to the withdrawal syndrome.

Chronic heavy drinking leads to physical dependence. In the UK, there are about 14 800 patients admitted each year to psychiatric hospitals for alcohol dependence and psychosis; brain damage and liver disease leading to cirrhosis are also common.

The physical withdrawal syndromes in humans range from a '*hangover*' to *epileptic fits* and the condition of '*delirium tremens*', in which the subject becomes agitated, confused and may have severe hallucinations. Alcohol withdrawal may require **diazepam** or, rarely, **clomethiazole** administration to prevent seizures. **Clonidine** may be helpful, but does not protect against fits. Maintenance of abstinence may be helped by daily **acamprosate** (mechanism unknown) or **disulfiram**, a drug that makes taking alcohol extremely unpleasant because it causes the accumulation of acetaldehyde.

Tobacco

Tobacco (nicotine) is a highly addictive drug that is responsible for more damage to health in the UK than all other drugs (including alcohol) combined. Nicotine increases alertness, decreases irritability and decreases skeletal muscle tone (because Renshaw cells are stimulated). Tolerance occurs to some effects of nicotine, notably the nausea and vomiting seen in non-tolerant subjects. The *toxicity of tobacco* is caused by the many chemicals in the smoke, some of which are known carcinogens. Serious diseases associated with chronic tobacco smoking include lung cancer, coronary heart disease and peripheral vascular disease. Smoking during pregnancy significantly reduces the birth weight of babies and increases perinatal mortality.

Withdrawal of tobacco causes a syndrome (lasting 2–3 weeks) that includes 'craving' for tobacco, irritability, hunger and often weight gain. These symptoms may be reduced by counselling in conjunction with **nicotine replacement therapy** (**NRT**) (e.g. chewing gum, nasal sprays, skin patches) or **bupropion** (amfebutamone), a drug that was originally developed as an antidepressant. After 1 year, about 20–30% of patients taking NRT or bupropion are not smoking, compared with only 10% of controls given a placebo.

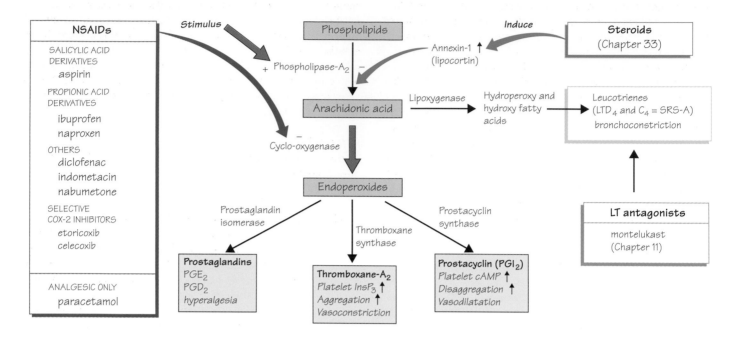

These drugs have *analgesic*, *antipyretic* and, at higher doses, *anti-inflammatory* actions. They are extensively used. In the UK, almost one-quarter of patients consulting their general practitioners have some form of 'rheumatic' complaint. These patients are frequently prescribed NSAIDs, and additional millions of **aspirin**, **paracetamol** and **ibuprofen** tablets are bought over the counter for the self-treatment of headaches, dental pain, various musculoskeletal disorders, etc. They are not effective in the treatment of visceral pain (e.g. myocardial infarction, renal colic, acute abdomen), which requires opioid analgesics. However, NSAIDs are effective in certain types of severe pain (e.g. bone cancer). Aspirin has important antiplatelet activity (Chapter 19).

The NSAIDs form a chemically diverse group (left), but they all have the ability to **inhibit cyclo-oxygenase** (**COX, ➡**), and the resulting inhibition of prostaglandin synthesis is largely responsible for their therapeutic effects. Unfortunately, the inhibition of prostaglandin synthesis in the gastric mucosa frequently results in *gastrointestinal damage* (dyspepsia, nausea and gastritis). More serious adverse effects include gastrointestinal bleeding and perforation. COX exists in the tissue as a constitutive isoform (COX-1) but, at sites of inflammation, cytokines stimulate the induction of a second isoform (COX-2). Inhibition of COX-2 is thought to be responsible for the anti-inflammatory actions of NSAIDs, whereas inhibition of COX-1 is responsible for their gastrointestinal toxicity. Most NSAIDs are somewhat selective for COX-1, but more recently selective COX-2 inhibitors have been introduced. **Celecoxib** and **etoricoxib** are selective COX-2 inhibitors that have similar efficacy to non-selective COX inhibitors, but the incidence of gastric perforation, obstruction and bleeding is reduced by at least 50%. However, these drugs are associated with an increased incidence of myocardial infarction and strokes. Non-selective NSAIDs may also be associated with a small increase in thrombo-embolic events.

Aspirin (acetylsalicylic acid) is the longest-standing NSAID and is an effective analgesic, with a duration of action of about 4 h. Aspirin is well absorbed orally. As it is a weak acid ($pK_a = 3.5$), the acid pH of the stomach keeps a large fraction of aspirin non-ionized and therefore promotes absorption in the stomach, although much aspirin is absorbed via the large surface area of the upper small intestine. The absorbed aspirin is hydrolysed by esterases in the blood and tissues to salicylate (which is active) and acetic acid. Most salicylate is converted in the liver to water-soluble conjugates that are rapidly excreted by the kidney. Alkalinization of the urine ionizes the salicylate and, because this reduces its tubular reabsorption, excretion is increased.

Aspirin was widely used in the treatment of inflammatory joint disease, but up to 50% of patients could not tolerate the adverse effects (nausea, vomiting, epigastric pain, tinnitus) caused by the high doses of soluble aspirin necessary to achieve an anti-inflammatory effect. For this reason, newer NSAIDs are generally preferred to treat the symptoms of inflammatory joint disease (pain, stiffness and swelling).

NSAIDs seem to have similar effectiveness. However, there is considerable patient variation in response and so it is impossible to know which drug will be effective in an individual, although 60% of patients will respond to any drug. Because the propionic acid derivatives (e.g. **ibuprofen**, **naproxen**) are associated with fewer serious adverse effects, these are often tried first.

Paracetamol has no significant anti-inflammatory action, but is widely used as a mild analgesic when pain has no inflammatory component. It is well absorbed orally and does not cause gastric irritation. It has the disadvantage that, in overdosage, serious hepatotoxicity is likely to occur (Chapters 4 and 45).

Mechanisms of action

Analgesic action. The analgesic action of NSAIDs is exerted both peripherally and centrally, but the peripheral actions predominate. The analgesic action is usually associated with the anti-inflammatory action of these agents, and results from the inhibition of prostaglandin synthesis in the inflamed tissues. Prostaglandins produce little pain by themselves, but potentiate the pain caused by other mediators of inflammation (e.g. histamine, bradykinin).

Anti-inflammatory action. The role of prostaglandins in inflammation is to produce vasodilatation and increased vascular permeability. However, inhibition of prostaglandin synthesis by NSAIDs attenuates rather than abolishes inflammation, because the drugs do not inhibit other mediators of inflammation. Nevertheless, the relatively modest anti-inflammatory actions of the NSAIDs give, to most patients with rheumatoid arthritis, some relief from pain, stiffness and swelling, but they do not alter the course of the disease.

Antipyretic action. NSAIDs do not reduce the normal body temperature or the elevated temperature in heat stroke, which is caused by hypothalamic malfunction. During fever, endogenous pyrogen (interleukin-1) is released from leucocytes and acts directly on the thermoregulatory centre in the hypothalamus to increase body temperature. This effect is associated with a rise in brain prostaglandins (which are pyrogenic). Aspirin prevents the temperature-raising effects of interleukin-1 by preventing the rise in brain prostaglandin levels.

Mechanism of action on cyclo-oxygenase. COX-1 and COX-2 enzymes possess a long channel, but this channel is wider in the COX-2 enzyme. Non-selective NSAIDs enter the channels in both enzymes and, except for aspirin, block them by binding via hydrogen bonds to an arginine residue halfway down. This reversibly inhibits the enzymes by preventing access for arachidonic acid. Aspirin is unique in that it acetylates the enzymes (at serine 530) and is therefore irreversible. Selective COX-2 inhibitors are generally more bulky molecules and can enter and block the channel in COX-2, but not the narrower channel of COX-1. **Paracetamol** acts at least partly by reducing cytoplasmic peroxide tone: peroxide is necessary to activate the haem COX enzyme to the ferryl form. In areas of acute inflammation, paracetamol is not very effective because neutrophils and monocytes produce high levels of H_2O_2 and lipid peroxide, which overcome the actions of the drug. However, paracetamol is an effective analgesic in conditions in which leucocyte infiltration is absent or low.

Adverse effects

Adverse effects of NSAIDs are common, partly because the drugs may be given in high doses for a long time and partly because they are widely used in elderly patients who are more susceptible to side-effects.

Gastrointestinal tract

In the stomach, COX-1 produces prostaglandins (PGE_2 and PGI_2) that stimulate mucus and bicarbonate secretion and cause vasodilatation, actions that protect the gastric mucosa (Chapter 12). Non-selective NSAIDs inhibit COX-1 and, because they reduce the cytoprotective effects of prostaglandins, they frequently cause serious upper gastrointestinal side-effects, including bleeding and ulceration. The newer selective COX-2 NSAIDs, e.g. **celecoxib**, are associated with a much lower incidence of gastrointestinal toxicity. However, COX-2 inhibitors are associated with a higher incidence of myocardial infarction and stroke than non-selective drugs, presumably because they do not inhibit the aggregation of platelets (which contain COX-1). For this reason, COX-2 inhibitors should not be used in patients with cardiovascular disease. **Misoprostol** is a PGE_1 derivative that is effective in preventing the gastrointestinal toxicity of NSAIDs. Its main indication is in patients with a history of peptic ulcer whose need for NSAID treatment is such that the analgesic cannot be withdrawn.

Nephrotoxicity

Prostaglandins PGE_2 and PGI_2 are powerful vasodilators synthesized in the renal medulla and glomeruli, respectively, and are involved in the control of renal blood flow and excretion of salt and water. Inhibition of renal prostaglandin synthesis may result in sodium retention, reduced renal blood flow and renal failure, especially in patients with conditions associated with vasoconstrictor catecholamines and angiotensin II release (e.g. congestive heart failure, cirrhosis). In addition, NSAIDs may cause interstitial nephritis and hyperkalaemia. Prolonged analgesic abuse over a period of years is associated with papillary necrosis and chronic renal failure.

Other adverse effects

These include bronchospasm, especially in asthmatics, skin rashes and other allergies.

Other NSAIDs

Propionic acids, such as **ibuprofen**, **fenbufen** and **naproxen**, are widely regarded as the drugs of first choice for the treatment of inflammatory joint disease, because they have the lowest incidence of side-effects. The selective COX-2 inhibitors **celecoxib** and **etoricoxib** have the lowest gastrointestinal toxicity but because of concerns about their cardiovascular safety, it is now considered unwise to use these drugs in preference to non-selective agents unless the patient is at serious risk of gastrointestinal ulceration or bleeding.

Diclofenac has similar actions to those of naproxen. It can be given by intravenous or deep intramuscular injection to prevent or treat post-operative pain.

Indometacin is one of the more effective agents, but has a higher incidence of adverse effects, including ulceration, gastric bleeding, headaches and dizziness. It may also cause blood dyscrasias.

Piroxicam has a long half-life and only requires the administration of a single daily dose. It may be associated with a particularly high incidence of gastrointestinal bleeding in the elderly.

Gout

Gout is characterized by the deposition of sodium urate crystals in the joints, causing painful arthritis. **Acute attacks** are treated with **diclofenac**, **indometacin** or other NSAIDs, but *not with aspirin*, which raises plasma urate levels at low doses by inhibiting uric acid secretion in the renal tubules. **Colchicine** is effective in gout. It binds to tubulin in leucocytes and prevents its polymerization into microtubules. This inhibits the phagocytic activity and migration of leucocytes to the areas of uric acid deposition, and hence reduces the inflammatory responses. However, colchicine causes nausea, vomiting, diarrhoea and abdominal pain.

Prophylactic treatment of gout

Allopurinol lowers plasma urate by inhibiting xanthine oxidase, the enzyme responsible for converting xanthine to uric acid. It is useful in patients with recurrent attacks of gout.

Uricosuric drugs, such as **sulfinpyrazone** and **probenecid**, inhibit renal tubular reabsorption of uric acid, increasing its excretion. Plenty of water should be taken to avoid the crystallization of urate in the urine. These drugs are less effective and more toxic than allopurinol. They are normally used in patients who cannot tolerate allopurinol.

33 Corticosteroids

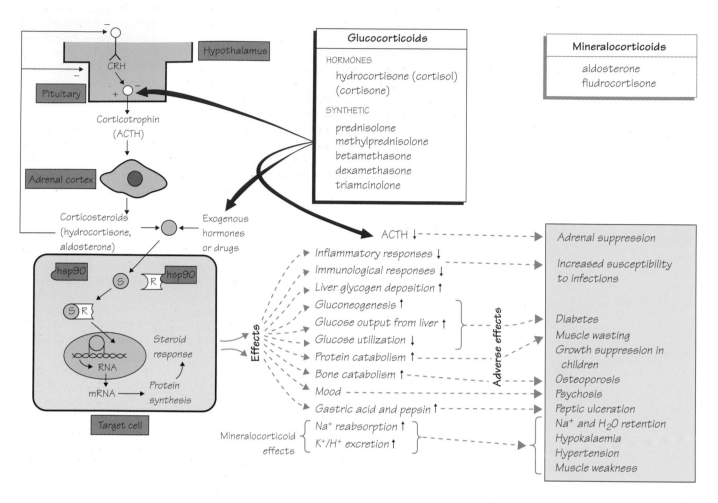

The adrenal cortex releases several steroid hormones into the circulation. They are divided by their actions into two classes:

1 Mineralocorticoids, mainly aldosterone in humans; have salt-retaining activity and are synthesized in the cells of the zona glomerulosa.

2 Glucocorticoids, mainly **cortisol** (hydrocortisone) in humans; affect carbohydrate and protein metabolism, but also have significant mineralocorticoid activity. They are synthesized in the cells of the zona fasciculata and zona reticularis.

The release of cortisol is controlled by a negative feedback mechanism involving the hypothalamus and anterior pituitary (upper figure, ▨). Low plasma cortisol levels result in the release of corticotrophin (adrenocorticotrophic hormone, ACTH), which stimulates cortisol synthesis and release by activating adenylyl cyclase. Cyclic adenosine monophosphate (cAMP) then activates protein kinase A, which phosphorylates and increases the activity of cholesterylester hydrolase, the rate-limiting step in steroid synthesis. Aldosterone release is affected by ACTH, but other factors (e.g. renin–angiotensin system, plasma potassium) are more important.

The steroids are examples of **gene-active** hormones. The steroid diffuses into the cells (lower figure, ⑤) where it binds to cytoplasmic glucocorticoid receptors (▯R). In the absence of cortisol, the receptor is inactivated by a heat-shock protein (▯hsp90). Cortisol triggers the release of hsp90 and the activated receptor (⑤R) enters the nucleus where it stimulates (or inhibits) the synthesis of proteins, which then produce the characteristic actions of the hormone (middle bottom).

The steroid **hormones** (**hydrocortisone** or **cortisone**) are given with a synthetic mineralocorticoid, usually **fludrocortisone** (top right), for replacement therapy in patients with adrenal insufficiency (e.g. in Addison's disease). For most therapeutic uses, **synthetic glucocorticoids** (top middle) have replaced the natural hormones, mainly because they have little or no salt-retaining activity.

Glucocorticoids (often **prednisolone**) are used to suppress inflammation, allergy and immune responses. Anti-inflammatory therapy is used in many diseases (e.g. rheumatoid arthritis, ulcerative colitis, bronchial asthma, severe inflammatory conditions of the eye and skin). Suppression of the immune system is of value in preventing rejection following tissue transplantation. Steroids are also used to suppress lymphopoiesis in patients with certain leukaemias and lymphomas.

Steroids can produce striking improvement in certain diseases, but high doses and prolonged use may cause **severe adverse effects** (right, ▨). These are usually predictable from the known actions of the drugs.

Corticotrophin-releasing hormone (CRH) is a 41-amino-acid polypeptide whose action is enhanced by arginine vasopressin (antidiuretic hormone, ADH). It is produced in the hypothalamus and reaches the adenohypophysis in the hypothalamo–hypophysial portal system, where it stimulates the release of corticotrophin.

Corticotrophin (ACTH) is processed from a large-molecular-weight precursor, pro-opiomelanocortin (POMC), present in corticotroph cells of the adenohypophysis; its main action is to stimulate the synthesis and release of *cortisol* (hydrocortisone). POMC also contains the sequences for *β-lipotropin* (β-LPH) and *β-endorphin*, which are concomitantly released into the blood. Corticotrophin is also believed to sensitize the zona glomerulosa to other stimuli that cause aldosterone release (i.e. low plasma Na$^+$, high plasma K$^+$, angiotensin II).

Glucocorticoids

Mechanisms of action

Cortisol (and synthetic glucocorticoids) diffuses into target cells and binds to a cytoplasmic glucocorticoid receptor belonging to the superfamily of steroid, thyroid (Chapter 35) and retinoid receptors. The activated receptor–glucocorticoid complex enters the nucleus and binds to steroid response elements on target DNA molecules. This either induces the synthesis of specific mRNA or represses genes by inhibiting transcription factors, e.g. nuclear factor κB (NFκB). For most clinical purposes, synthetic glucocorticoids are used because they have a higher affinity for the receptor, are less rapidly inactivated and have little or no salt-retaining properties.

Hydrocortisone is used (i) orally for replacement therapy; (ii) intravenously in shock and status asthmaticus; and (iii) topically (e.g. ointments in eczema, enemas in ulcerative colitis).

Prednisolone is the drug most widely given orally in inflammatory and allergic diseases.

Betamethasone and **dexamethasone** are very potent and have no salt-retaining actions. This makes them especially useful for high-dose therapy in conditions, such as cerebral oedema, where water retention would be a disadvantage.

Beclometasone dipropionate and **budesonide** pass membranes poorly and are more active topically than when given orally. They are used in asthma (as an aerosol) and topically in severe eczema to provide a local anti-inflammatory action with minimal systemic effects.

Triamcinolone is used in severe asthma and by intra-articular injection for local inflammation of joints.

Effects

Glucocorticoids influence most cells in the body.

Metabolic effects Glucocorticoids are essential for life, their most important action being to facilitate the conversion of protein to glycogen. Glucocorticoids inhibit protein synthesis and stimulate protein catabolism to amino acids. Gluconeogenesis, glycogen deposition and glucose release from the liver are stimulated, but peripheral glucose uptake is inhibited. During fasting, glucocorticoids are vital to prevent (possibly fatal) hypoglycaemia.

Anti-inflammatory and immunosuppressive effects Corticosteroids have profound anti-inflammatory effects and are widely used for this purpose. They suppress all phases of the inflammatory response, including the early swelling, redness and pain, and the later proliferative changes seen in chronic inflammation. Inflammation is suppressed by several mechanisms. Circulating immunocompetent cells and macrophages are reduced and the formation of pro-inflammatory medi-

ators, such as prostaglandins, leucotrienes and platelet activating factor (PAF), is inhibited. Steroids produce these latter effects by stimulating the synthesis in leucocytes of a protein (annexin-1) that inhibits phospholipase A$_2$. This enzyme, located in the cell membrane, is activated in damaged cells and is responsible for the formation of arachidonic acid, the precursor of many inflammatory mediators (Chapter 32). Corticosteroids also suppress the genes encoding phospholipase A$_2$, cyclo-oxygenase-2 (COX-2) and the interleukin-2 (IL-2) receptor. These genes are normally switched on by NFκB, but steroids induce the synthesis of IκB, which binds to NFκB and inhibits it by preventing its entry into the nucleus.

Glucocorticoids depress monocyte/macrophage function and decrease circulating thymus-derived lymphocytes (T-cells), especially helper T$_4$ lymphocytes. The release of IL-1 and IL-2 (necessary to activate and stimulate lymphocyte proliferation) is inhibited. The transport of lymphocytes to the site of antigenic stimulation and the production of antibody are also inhibited.

Adverse effects

Glucocorticoids produce many adverse effects, especially with the high doses required for anti-inflammatory activity. (Similar effects are produced by the excess corticosteroids secreted in Cushing's syndrome.)

Metabolic effects High doses quickly cause a rounded, plethoric face (moon face), and fat is redistributed from the extremities to the trunk and face. Purple striae and a tendency to bruise develop. Disturbed carbohydrate metabolism leads to hyperglycaemia and occasionally diabetes. Protein loss from skeletal muscles causes wasting and weakness. This cannot be remedied by dietary protein because protein synthesis is inhibited. An increase in bone catabolism may cause osteoporosis. **Bisphosphonates** (e.g. **etidronate**, **alendronate**) are incorporated into the bone matrix and accumulate in the osteoclasts when they resorb bone. This results in inhibition and apoptosis of the osteoclasts and reduction of bone resorption. Bisphosphonates can be used for the prevention and treatment of corticosteroid-induced osteoporosis and to treat osteoporosis in postmenopausal women (Chapter 34).

Fluid retention, hypokalaemia and hypertension These may occur with compounds that have significant mineralocorticoid activity. Thus, hydrocortisone (and cortisone) are generally used only for replacement therapy in adrenal insufficiency.

Adrenal suppression Steroid therapy suppresses corticotrophin secretion and this eventually leads to adrenal atrophy. It may take 6–12 months for normal adrenal function to recover once therapy is stopped. Because the patient's response to stress is suppressed, additional steroid must be administered in times of severe stress (e.g. surgery, infection). Steroid therapy must be withdrawn very gradually, because abrupt withdrawal causes adrenal insufficiency.

Infections There is increased susceptibility to infections, which may progress unrecognized because the natural indicators of infection are inhibited.

Other complications These include psychosis, cataracts, glaucoma, peptic ulceration and the reactivation of nascent infections (e.g. tuberculosis).

Mineralocorticoids

Fludrocortisone is given with hydrocortisone in adrenal insufficiency (e.g. Addison's disease or following adrenalectomy) because the latter drug does not possess sufficient salt-retaining activity.

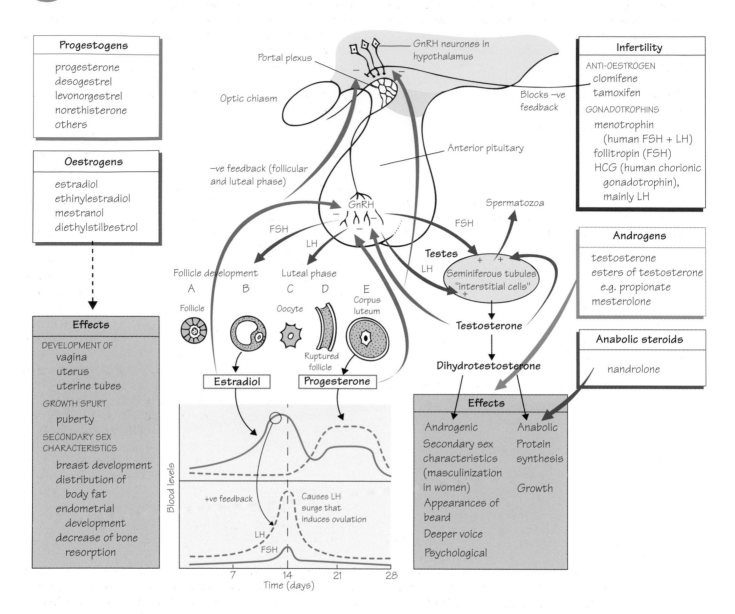

The ovaries and testes, in addition to producing gametes, also secrete hormones (mainly **oestrogens** and **androgens**, respectively). The secretion of oestrogens (mainly **estradiol**) and androgens (mainly **testosterone**) requires **gonadotrophins** (luteinizing hormone, LH; and follicle-stimulating hormone, FSH), which are hormones released from the anterior pituitary (middle top). The release of LH and FSH is, in turn, controlled by the hypothalamus (top, ☐), which releases pulses of gonadotrophin-releasing hormone (GnRH).

In the **testes** (right, ⬭), spermatozoa are produced in the seminiferous tubules by a process requiring both FSH and *testosterone*, the latter hormone being synthesized in the interstitial cells in response to LH. Testosterone causes the changes that occur in the normal male at puberty (bottom right, shaded). **Androgens** (middle right) are used mainly for replacement therapy in castrated males or in males who are hypogonadal either because of pituitary or testicular disease. **Testosterone** is rapidly inactivated by the liver following oral administration,

but synthetic androgens (e.g. **mesterolone**) are active orally. **Anabolic steroids** (bottom right) have relatively little androgenic activity and are used to try to increase protein synthesis after major surgery and in chronic debilitating disease. The main adverse effects of androgens and, to a lesser extent, the anabolic steroids are masculinization in women and prepubertal children and the suppression of FSH and LH.

In the **ovary**, FSH (and LH) stimulates follicular development (middle left, A–B) and **estradiol** synthesis by the granulosa cells of the follicle. In the early follicular phase, the low estradiol level in the blood (middle left) exerts a negative feedback effect on FSH, ensuring that only the dominant follicle ripens. Midway through the cycle, estradiol levels are high and this has a positive feedback effect on LH secretion, leading to the 'LH surge' (bottom left) that causes ovulation. These feedback effects of estradiol are exerted on the hypothalamus (changing the amount of GnRH secreted) and the pituitary gland (altering its response to GnRH). The ruptured follicle (D) develops into the corpus luteum (E), which secretes oestrogen and progesterone (middle left) until the end of the cycle. During the follicular phase of the cycle, oestrogen stimulates endometrial proliferation. In the luteal phase, increased progesterone release stimulates the maturation and glandular development of the endometrium, which is then shed in the process of menstruation.

Oestrogens (middle left) have many effects (bottom left, shaded).

GnRH (**gonadorelin**) is a decapeptide that stimulates FSH and LH release from the anterior pituitary gland. Pulsatile infusions of GnRH are used to treat hypothalamic hypogonadism.

LH and **FSH** are glycoprotein hormones produced by the anterior pituitary. They regulate gonadal function.

Infertility

In anovulatory women, infertility may be overcome provided that the ovary is capable of producing mature ova and the appropriate steroids.

Clomifene and **tamoxifen** are anti-oestrogens. They work by inhibiting the feedback inhibition of oestrogens in the hypothalamus and so increase FSH and LH release.

Gonadotrophins are used in women who lack appropriate pituitary function or do not respond to clomifene therapy. Treatment starts with daily injections of **menotrophin** (LH and FSH in equal amounts) or **recombinant human follitropin** (FSH), followed by one or two large doses of **chorionic gonadotrophin** (mainly LH) to induce ovulation. Multiple births occur in 20–30% of pregnancies after treatment. In men with hypogonadotrophic hypogonadism, both gonadotrophins are sometimes given to stimulate spermatogenesis and androgen release.

Testosterone

The most important androgen in humans is testosterone. About 2% of testosterone in the plasma is free, and in the skin, prostate, seminal vesicles and epididymis it is converted to dihydrotestosterone. Androgen deficiency is usually treated with intramuscular depot injections of testosterone propionate.

Effects At puberty, androgens cause development of the secondary sexual characteristics in the male. In the adult male, large doses suppress the release of gonadotrophins and cause some atrophy of the interstitial tissue and tubules of the testes. In women, androgens cause changes, many of which are similar to those seen in the prepubertal male.

Oestrogens

Estradiol is the main oestrogen released by the human ovary. Synthetic oestrogens are more effective following oral administration.

Adverse effects (see 'Oral contraceptives' below) The continuous administration of oestrogens for prolonged periods can cause abnormal endometrial hyperplasia and abnormal bleeding patterns, and is associated with an increased incidence of endometrial carcinoma. When a progestogen is given with the oestrogen, there is a decreased incidence of ovarian and endometrial cancers. Thus, women taking HRT must also take a progestogen unless they have had a hysterectomy.

Progestogens

Progestogens are used for hormonal contraception and for producing long-term ovarian suppression for other purposes (e.g. dysmenorrhoea,

They are used for hormone replacement therapy (HRT) in primary hypogonadism and in postmenopausal women to prevent hot flushes, atrophic vaginitis and osteoporosis. They are also used in a number of menstrual disorders (e.g. spasmodic dysmenorrhoea) and, in combination with progestogens, as contraceptives. **Progestogens** (top left) are used mainly for hormonal contraception. Sex hormones and antagonists are used in the treatment of certain cancers (Chapter 44).

---

endometriosis, hirsutism and bleeding disorders) when oestrogens are contraindicated.

Oral contraceptives

Combination pills contain oestrogen, usually ethinylestradiol, and a progestogen. They are taken for 20–21 days and discontinued for the following 6–7 days to allow menstruation to occur.

Progestogen-only pills contain a low dose of progestogen (e.g. norethisterone) and are taken continuously.

Enzyme-inducing drugs, e.g. phenobarbital, carbamazepine, phenytoin and especially rifampicin, may cause failure of contraception.

Mechanism of action. Combination pills act by feedback inhibition on the hypothalamus to suppress GnRH and hence plasma gonadotrophin secretion, thereby blocking ovulation. These drugs also produce an endometrium that is unreceptive to implantation, alter Fallopian tube motility and change the composition of cervical mucus. These latter effects are also produced by progestogen-only pills and appear to be the basis of their contraceptive actions, because they block ovulation in only about 25% of women. Menstruation often ceases initially with progestogens, but usually returns with prolonged administration. However, the length and duration of bleeding are very variable.

Adverse effects. *Non-life-threatening* side-effects that occur with both combination pills and progestogens include breakthrough bleeding, weight gain, changes in libido, breast soreness, headache and nausea. Combination pills may also cause hirsutism, vaginal yeast infections and depression. About 20–30% of women will experience some of these effects, and 10–15% will stop taking the pill because of them. The overall incidence of side-effects is lower with progestogen-only pills, but breakthrough bleeding and irregular menses are major complaints with these drugs.

Serious side-effects are rare. They include cholestatic jaundice and a slightly greater incidence of thromboembolic disease, for which the oestrogen is apparently responsible. Combined pills containing gestodene and desogestrel are associated with a slightly higher incidence of thromboembolism. However, the absolute risk of thromboembolism is very small (about 25 incidents per 100 000 women per year). A history of thromboembolism, cigarette smoking, hypertension and diabetes increases the thromboembolic risk of oral contraception. Oral contraceptives are probably associated with a small increase in the risk of breast cancer.

Emergency contraception Emergency contraception can be produced up to 3 days after unprotected intercourse by giving a single high dose of **levonorgestrel**.

Therapeutic termination of pregnancy Progesterone supports endometrial nidation of the fertilized ovum, and the progesterone antagonist, **mifepristone**, is highly effective in terminating early pregnancy (up to 63 days' gestation) when used with a prostaglandin cervical ripening agent (e.g. gemeprost pessaries). The main adverse effects are pain and bleeding.

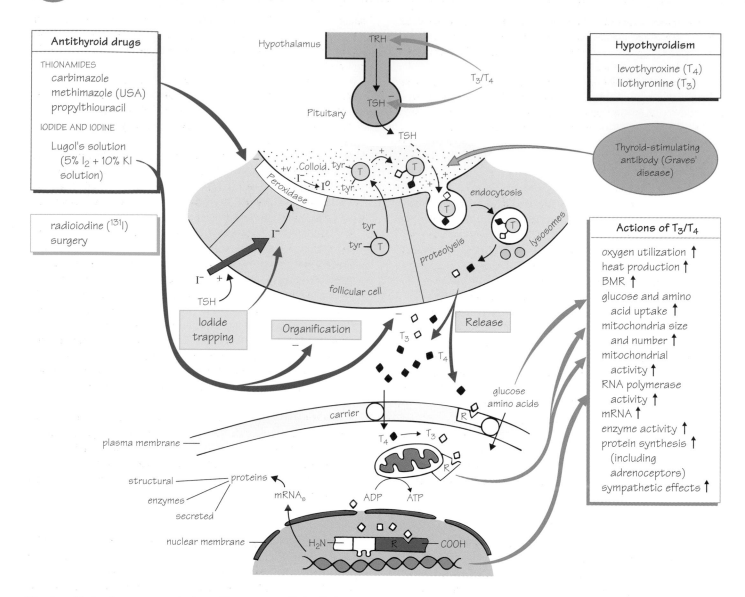

The thyroid gland secretes two iodinated hormones called **triiodothyronine** (T_3) and **thyroxine** (**levothyroxine**, tetraiodothyronine, T_4), which are responsible for the optimal growth, development, function and maintenance of body tissues. Another hormone, **calcitonin**, is produced by the parafollicular cells and is involved in the regulation of calcium metabolism.

The synthesis of T_3 and T_4 requires **iodine**, which is normally ingested (as iodide) in the diet. An active, *thyrotrophin*-dependent pump (➡) concentrates the **iodide** (I^-) in the follicular cells (centre figure shaded orange) where, at the apical boundary, it is rapidly oxidized by peroxidase to the more reactive **iodine** (I^0). The iodine reacts with tyrosine residues present in thyroglobulin ('organification', ⓣ), and units of T_3 (◇) and T_4 (◆) are formed. The thyroglobulin containing these iodothyronines is stored in the follicles as colloid (□).

The release of T_3 and T_4 is controlled by a negative feedback system (top figure). When the circulating levels of T_3 and T_4 fall, **thyrotrophin** (**thyroid-stimulating hormone, TSH**) is released from the anterior pituitary gland and stimulates the transport of colloid

(by endocytosis) into the follicular cells. Then, the colloid droplets fuse with lysosomes (◯), and protease enzymes degrade the thyroglobulin, releasing T_3 (◇) and T_4 (◆) into the circulation. Both thyroid hormones act on **receptors** (**R**) in the plasma membrane and on intracellular receptors (bottom figure) to produce a variety of actions (right).

Thyroid hyperfunction and hypofunction occur in about 2% of the population and, together with diabetes mellitus (2–3% of the population), are the most common endocrine disorders. In **Graves' disease**, hyperthyroidism is produced by an IgG antibody that causes prolonged activation of the TSH receptors and results in excessive secretion of T_3 and T_4. Thyroid activity can be reduced with drugs that decrease hormone synthesis (left), or by the destruction of the gland with radiation (using ^{131}I) or surgery. Hyperthyroidism often causes increased sympathetic effects, which can be blocked with β-adrenoceptor antagonists (e.g. propranolol). Graves' disease is often associated with ophthalmopathy, which is often difficult to control, and may be a distinct organ-specific autoimmune disease.

Primary hypothyroidism (**myxoedema**) probably results in most cases from a cell-mediated immune response directed against the thyroid follicular cells. **Levothyroxine** is the drug of choice for replacement therapy (top right).

Thyrotrophin-releasing hormone (**TRH**) is a tripeptide synthesized in the hypothalamus and transported in the capillaries of the pituitary portal venous system to the pituitary gland, where it stimulates TSH synthesis and release.

Thyrotrophin (**TSH**) is a glycoprotein hormone that is released from the pituitary gland (adenohypophysis). It activates receptors on the follicular cells and increases cyclic adenosine monophosphate (cAMP), which stimulates the synthesis and release of hormones from the thyroid gland. In hypothyroidism or, rarely, iodine deficiency, abnormally high levels of TSH result in the enlargement of the thyroid gland (goitre).

T_3 **and** T_4. Triiodothyronine and thyroxine (tetraiodothyronine) enter the circulation, where they are transported largely bound to plasma proteins (99.5% and 99.95%, respectively). The thyroid only contributes about 20% of the unbound circulating T_3, the remainder being produced by the *peripheral conversion* of T_4 to T_3. T_4 may also be deiodinated to inactive reverse T_3 (rT_3) according to the demands of the tissues. T_4 seems to be mainly a prohormone of T_3.

Actions. The mechanisms of action of the thyroid hormones are not fully understood, but are thought to involve high-affinity binding sites (receptors) in the *plasma membrane*, *mitochondria* and *nucleus*. These receptor–hormone interactions result in a variety of effects, including increased protein synthesis and an increase in energy metabolism. Most **receptors** are intracellular. The nuclear receptors for T_3 (and steroids and vitamin D) are encoded by a superfamily of genes related to the *cis*-oncogenes. Free T_3/T_4 enters the cell by a carrier mechanism and most T_4 is converted to T_3 (or rT_3), which binds to the C-terminus of the receptor and induces a conformational change in its DNA binding site. This permits the activated receptor to interact with a thyroid hormone regulatory element in the target DNA molecules. Hence, gene transcription and protein synthesis are stimulated or repressed.

Hyperthyroidism (thyrotoxicosis)
The basal metabolic rate is increased, causing heat intolerance, arrhythmias and increased appetite. The skin is warm and moist. There is increased nervousness and hyperkinesia. Sympathetic overactivity causes tachycardia, sweating and tremor. Angina and high-output heart failure may occur. The upper eyelids are retracted, causing a wide stare.

Traditionally, young patients have been treated with antithyroid drugs and, if the condition relapses, subtotal thyroidectomy. Patients over about 40 years of age have been given radioiodine therapy. Nowadays, young patients may be given ^{131}I, and carbimazole may be given long-term.

Antithyroid drugs
Thionamides possess a thiocarbamide group (S=C–N) that is essential for their activity. They prevent the synthesis of thyroid hormones by competitively inhibiting the peroxidase-catalysed reactions necessary for iodine organification. They also block the coupling of iodotyrosine, especially diiodothyronine formation. Thionamides may be immuno-suppressive, but this is controversial. All the antithyroid drugs are administered orally and are accumulated in the thyroid gland. Their onset of action is delayed until the preformed hormones are depleted, a process that may take 3–4 weeks.

Carbimazole is rapidly converted to methimazole *in vivo*. The aim is to render the patient euthyroid and then to give a reduced dose for maintenance. It is often possible to cease treatment after 1 or 2 years. Side-effects include rashes and, rarely, agranulocytosis (warn patients to report a sore throat).

Propylthiouracil is usually reserved for patients who are intolerant to carbimazole. It is associated with a higher incidence of agranulocytosis (0.4%) than carbimazole (0.1%). In addition to inhibiting hormone synthesis, propylthiouracil also inhibits the peripheral deiodination of T_4 and perhaps has an immunosuppressive action.

Iodides have several poorly understood actions on the thyroid. They inhibit organification and hormone release. In addition, iodide decreases the size and vascularity of the hyperplastic gland, effects which are useful in the preparation of patients for thyroidectomy. In 'pharmacological' doses, the main effect of iodides is to inhibit hormone release (possibly by inhibition of thyroglobulin proteolysis) and, because thyrotoxic symptoms are reduced relatively quickly (2–7 days), iodine is valuable in the treatment of **thyrotoxic crisis** ('thyroid storm') – a life-threatening acute exacerbation of all the symptoms of thyrotoxicosis. Iodine cannot be used for the long-term treatment of hyperthyroidism because its antithyroid action tends to diminish.

Propranolol or **atenolol** can reduce the heart rate and other sympathetic manifestations of hyperthyroidism and provide partial relief of symptoms until full control is achieved with carbimazole. It is useful in the preoperative preparation of patients undergoing thyroidectomy. Propranolol is also used together with hydrocortisone, iodine and carbimazole in '**thyroid storm**'.

Hypothyroidism
Tiredness and lethargy are the most common symptoms of hypothyroidism. Other effects include depression of the basal metabolic rate, appetite and cardiac output. Low-output heart failure may occur. The skin is dry. Thyroid hormone deprivation in early life results in irreversible mental retardation and dwarfism (cretinism) and, to prevent this, all newborn infants are screened and replacement therapy is given from birth.

Replacement therapy
Levothyroxine (thyroxine) administered orally is the treatment of choice. Synthetic T_4 is the sodium salt of levothyroxine (L-thyroxine). Its effects are delayed until the plasma protein and tissue binding sites are occupied. Treatment is assessed by monitoring plasma TSH levels, which fall to normal when the optimum dose is achieved.

Liothyronine is the sodium salt of T_3 and, because it is less protein-bound, it acts more quickly than T_4. The main use of T_3 is in hypothyroid coma, when it is given (together with hydrocortisone) by intravenous injection.

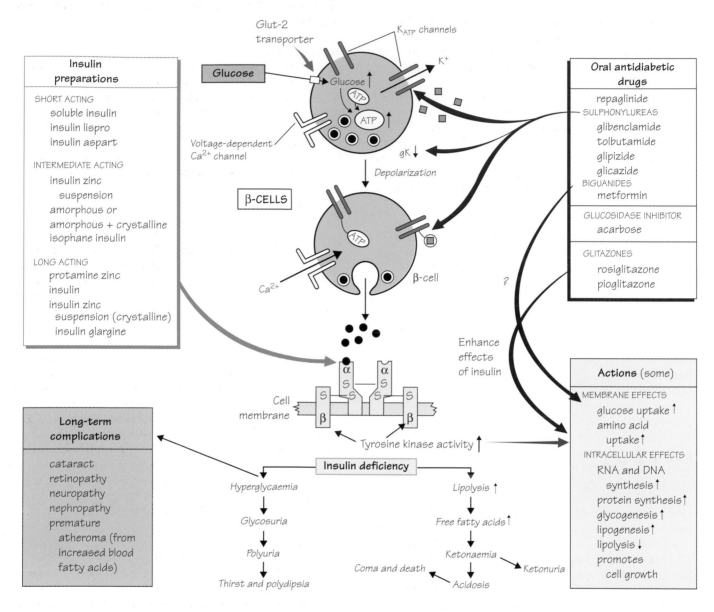

Insulin is a hormone secreted by the β-cells of the islets of Langerhans in the pancreas (top). Various stimuli **release** insulin (●) from storage granules (◉) in the β-cells, but the most potent stimulus is a rise in plasma glucose (hyperglycaemia). Insulin binds to specific **receptors** (middle) in the cell membranes, initiating a number of actions (bottom right, shaded), including an increase in glucose uptake by muscle, liver and adipose tissue.

In **diabetes mellitus**, there is a relative or total absence of insulin, which causes reduced glucose uptake by insulin-sensitive tissues and has serious consequences (middle bottom). Lipolysis and muscle proteolysis result in weight loss and weakness. The blood levels of free fatty acids and glycerol rise. An excess of acetyl-CoA is produced in the liver and converted to *acetoacetic acid*, which is then either reduced to *β-hydroxybutyric acid* or decarboxylated to *acetone*. These 'ketone bodies' accumulate in the blood, causing an acidosis (ketoacidosis).

About 25% of diabetics have a severe deficiency of insulin. This **type**

I, or **insulin-dependent**, **diabetes** is associated with human leucocyte antigens and immunologically selective β-cell destruction. In these patients, *ketosis* is common and insulin is required. Various **insulin preparations** (top left) and **regimens** are used. There is evidence that metabolic control early in the course of the disease may prevent or delay the onset of diabetic complications (bottom left, shaded). In **type II**, or **non-insulin-dependent**, **diabetes** the aetiology is unknown, but a strong genetic component is present. There is a resistance to circulating insulin, which does, however, protect the patient from ketosis. The number of insulin receptors is reduced, and this is often associated with obesity. Loss of weight (diet and exercise) reduces insulin 'resistance' and controls about one-third of type II diabetics. Another one-third of type II diabetics are controlled by diet together with **oral antidiabetic drugs** (top right). The **sulphonylureas** (▪) and **repaglinide** close K$_{ATP}$ channels (middle), causing depolarization of the β-cells and increased insulin release. **Acarbose** delays the absorption of glucose following a meal. The **glitazones** improve sensitivity to insulin. Type II diabetics not controlled by diet and oral antidiabetic drugs require insulin injections. These tend to be the thinner patients who lack the first-phase insulin response.

Insulin

Insulin is a polypeptide containing 51 amino acids arranged in two chains (A and B) linked by disulphide bridges. A precursor, called proinsulin, is hydrolysed inside storage granules to form insulin and a residual C-peptide. The granules store insulin as crystals containing zinc and insulin.

Insulin release. Glucose is the most potent stimulus for insulin release from islet β-cells. There is a continuous basal secretion with surges at feeding times. The β-cells possess K^+ channels that are regulated by intracellular adenosine triphosphate (ATP) (K_{ATP} channels). When the blood glucose increases, more glucose enters the β-cells and its metabolism results in an increase in intracellular ATP, which closes the K_{ATP} channels. The resulting depolarization of the β-cell initiates an influx of Ca^{2+} ions through voltage-sensitive Ca^{2+} channels and this triggers insulin release.

Insulin receptors. Insulin receptors are membrane-spanning glycoproteins consisting of two α subunits and two β subunits linked covalently by disulphide bonds. After insulin binds to the α subunit, the insulin–receptor complex enters the cell, where the insulin is destroyed by lysosomal enzymes. The internalization of the insulin–receptor complex underlies the *downregulation* of receptors that is produced by high levels of insulin (e.g. in obese subjects). The binding of insulin to the receptors activates the tyrosine kinase activity of the β subunit and initiates a complex chain of reactions that lead to the effects of insulin.

Insulin preparations

Most diabetics in the UK are now treated with human insulin. Insulin is administered by subcutaneous injection and its rate of *absorption* can be decreased either by *increasing the particle size* (i.e. crystals are absorbed slower than amorphous) or by *complexing the insulin with zinc or protamine.*

Short-acting insulins

Soluble insulin is a simple solution of insulin. (Onset 30 min, peak activity 2–4 h, subsides by 8 h.) It can be administered intravenously in hyperglycaemic emergencies, but its effects last for only 30 min by this route. **Insulin lispro** and **insulin aspart** are insulin analogues that have a faster onset and shorter action than soluble insulin. This is because, unlike regular insulin, they do not self-associate to form dimers. A human insulin preparation for inhalation is available for patients who cannot be given injections.

Intermediate- and long-acting insulins

Isophane insulin is a complex of protamine and insulin. After injection, proteolytic enzymes degrade the protamine and the insulin is absorbed. **Biphasic fixed mixtures** contain various proportions of soluble and isophane insulin (e.g. 30% soluble and 70% isophane). The soluble component gives a rapid onset and the isophane insulin prolongs the action. **Insulin zinc suspension (crystalline)** is a suspension of poorly soluble insulin zinc crystals that has a duration of up to 35 h. **Insulin zinc suspension** is a mixture of amorphous (30%) and crystalline (70%) insulin zinc, the latter prolonging the duration of this preparation.

Protamine zinc insulin is a suspension of insulin with both zinc and protamine. It has a long duration but is not used often because it binds to soluble insulin if they are mixed together in the same syringe.

Insulin glargine is soluble at acid pH, but precipitates in the more neutral tissue pH. It has a long 'peakless' activity (11–12 h) and is given once a day.

Adverse effects

Hypoglycaemia caused by insulin overdose or inadequate calorific intake is the most common and most serious complication of insulin treatment. When severe, coma and death will occur if the patient is not treated with glucose (intravenously if patient is unconscious).

Insulin antibodies. All insulins are immunogenic to some extent (bovine most), but immunological resistance to insulin is rare.

Lipohypertrophy is common with all preparations of insulin, but local allergic reactions at the injection site are now very rare.

Insulin regimens

Most type I diabetic patients use a regimen involving a short-acting insulin mixed with intermediate-acting insulin injected subcutaneously twice daily, before breakfast and before the evening meal. More demanding, intensive control regimens, designed to produce nearnormoglycaemia, reduce diabetic complications (left, shaded). One such regimen is an injection of intermediate-acting insulin, to provide a background level of insulin, and soluble insulin three times a day before meals.

Oral antidiabetic drugs

Sulphonylureas are indicated in patients (especially those near their ideal weight) in whom diet fails to control the hyperglycaemia – although in about 30% control is not achieved with these drugs. These agents stimulate insulin release from the pancreatic islets and so the patient must have *partially functional β-cells* for these drugs to be of use. **Glipizide** and **glicazide** have relatively short half-lives and are commonly tried first. **Glibenclamide** has a longer duration of action and can be given once daily. However, there is more chance of hypoglycaemia, and glibenclamide should be avoided in patients at risk from hypoglycaemia (e.g. the elderly). These patients may be more safely given **tolbutamide**, which has the shortest duration of action.

Adverse effects

Gastrointestinal disturbances and rashes occur, but are rare. Hypoglycaemia and hypoglycaemic coma may be induced by longer-acting drugs, *especially in elderly patients*. Sulphonylureas are contraindicated in severe (especially ketotic) hyperglycaemia, surgery and major illness, when insulin should be given.

Repaglinide has a rapid onset and short duration of action. It is taken at the onset of a meal to provide a surge of insulin release during digestion with a reduced risk of interprandial hypoglycaemia.

Biguanides. **Metformin** reduces hepatic glucose production and acts peripherally to increase glucose uptake. As it does not increase insulin release, it rarely causes hypoglycaemia.

Acarbose inhibits intestinal α-glycosidases, delaying the digestion of starch and sucrose. It is taken with meals and lowers the postprandial increase of blood glucose. Its main side-effect is flatulence.

Glitazones (thiazolidinediones). These drugs increase sensitivity to insulin by binding to the nuclear peroxisome proliferator-activated receptor gamma (PPAR-γ) and, by derepression, increase transcription of certain insulin-sensitive genes. They are given alone or in combination with metformin or sulphonylureas in patients who cannot tolerate metformin and sulphonylurea combinations.

37 Antibacterial drugs that inhibit nucleic acid synthesis: sulphonamides, trimethoprim, quinolones and nitroimidazoles

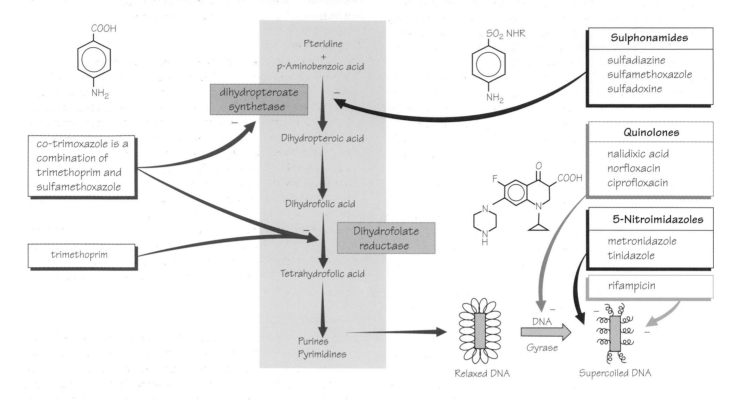

The sulphonamides were the first drugs found to be effective in the treatment of systemic infections. However, they are now rarely used for bacterial infections because of the development of more effective agents that are less toxic. Also, many organisms have developed **resistance** to sulphonamides. Their principal use alone is in the treatment of urinary tract infections caused by sensitive Gram-positive or Gram-negative organisms.*

There are many sulphonamides, and a few examples are given together with their general structure (top right). They are structural analogues of *p*-aminobenzoic acid (top left), which is essential for folic acid synthesis in bacteria. The **selective toxicity** of the sulphonamides depends on the fact that mammalian cells take up folate supplied in the diet, but susceptible bacteria lack this ability and must synthesize folate. Sulphonamides competitively inhibit the enzyme dihydropteroate synthetase ( ), and prevent the production of folate required for the synthesis of DNA. The sulphonamides are bacteriostatic agents. Their most important side-effects are rashes (common), renal failure and blood dyscrasias.

Trimethoprim (bottom left) acts on the same metabolic pathway as sulphonamides, but is an inhibitor of dihydrofolate reductase ( ). It is selectively toxic because its affinity for the bacterial enzyme is 50 000 times greater than its affinity for the human enzyme. Trimethoprim is widely used in urinary tract infections. A combination of trimethoprim and sulfamethoxazole (**co-trimoxazole**, left) may produce a synergistic action and increased activity against certain bacteria. Co-trimoxazole has an important use in the treatment of *Pneumocystis jiroveci* (*Pneumocystis carinii*) pneumonia.

The **quinolones** (middle right) inhibit DNA gyrase ( ), an enzyme that compresses bacterial DNA into supercoils. To fit the comparatively long, double-stranded DNA into the bacterial cell, it is arranged in loops (relaxed DNA, bottom right), which are then shortened by supercoiling. The quinolones are bactericidal because they inhibit resealing of the DNA strands that are opened in the supercoiling process. Eukaryotic cells do not contain DNA gyrase. **Ciprofloxacin** is a broad-spectrum antibacterial agent. Important properties of the quinolones are their good penetration into tissues and cells (cf. penicillins), their effectiveness when given orally and their relatively low toxicity.

The **5-nitroimidazoles**, e.g. **metronidazole** (bottom right), have a very wide spectrum and are active against anaerobic bacteria and some protozoa (Chapter 43). The drug diffuses into the organism where the nitro group is reduced. During this reduction process, chemically reactive intermediates are formed that inhibit DNA synthesis and/or damage DNA, impairing its function.

Rifampicin prevents RNA transcription in many bacteria by inhibiting DNA-dependent RNA polymerase (bottom right). Resistance to rifampicin quickly develops but, in combination with other drugs, it is important in the treatment of tuberculosis (Chapter 39).

* Bacteria are classified by their shape (cocci are spherical, bacilli are rod-shaped), and many also by whether (Gram-positive) or not (Gram-negative) they remain stained with methyl violet after washing with acetone. The retention or not of methyl violet reflects important differences in the bacterial cell walls.

Selective toxicity

The use of chemicals to try to eradicate parasites, bacteria, viruses or cancer cells in the body is called chemotherapy. It depends on the drugs being selectively toxic, i.e. toxic to the cells of the parasite, but not (too) toxic to the human host. Bacterial cells have many biochemical differences from human cells, and some antibacterial drugs are strikingly non-toxic to humans. However, because cancer cells are so similar to normal cells, most anticancer drugs show little selective toxicity and therefore produce serious adverse effects (Chapter 44).

Bacteriostatic agents inhibit bacterial growth, whereas **bactericidal agents** actually kill the organism. This distinction is not usually important clinically, as host defence mechanisms are involved in the final elimination of bacterial pathogens. An exception is the treatment of infections in immunocompromised patients (AIDS, corticosteroids, anticancer and immunosuppressant drugs), when a bactericidal agent should be used.

Resistance to antimicrobial drugs can be acquired or innate. In the latter case, an entire bacterial species may be resistant to a drug before its introduction. For example, *Pseudomonas aeruginosa* has always been resistant to **flucloxacillin**. More serious clinically is **acquired resistance**, where bacteria that were once sensitive to a drug become resistant. Mechanisms responsible for resistance to antimicrobial drugs include the following:

1 Inactivating enzymes that destroy the drug, e.g. β-lactamases produced by many staphylococci inactivate most penicillins and many cephalosporins.

2 Decreased drug accumulation. Tetracycline resistance occurs where the bacterial cell membrane becomes impermeable to the drug or there is increased efflux.

3 Alteration of binding sites. Aminoglycosides and erythromycin bind to bacterial ribosomes and inhibit protein synthesis. In resistant organisms, the sites of drug binding may be modified so that they no longer have affinity for the drugs.

4 Development of alternative metabolic pathways. Bacteria can become resistant to sulphonamides and trimethoprim because they produce modified dihydropteroate synthetase and dihydrofolate reductase enzymes, respectively, which have little or no affinity for the drugs.

Antibiotic-resistant bacterial populations can develop in several ways:

1 Selection. Within a population there will be some bacteria with acquired resistance. The drug then eliminates the sensitive organisms and the resistant forms proliferate.

2 Transferred resistance. Here, the gene that codes for the resistance mechanism is transferred from one organism to another. The antibiotic resistance genes may be carried in **plasmids**, which are small autonomously replicating extrachromosomal pieces of DNA within the bacteria. The plasmids (and therefore antibiotic resistance) can be transferred from one organism to another by *conjugation* (the formation of a tube between the organisms). Many Gram-negative and some Gram-positive bacteria can conjugate. In *transduction*, plasmid DNA is enclosed in a bacterial virus (bacteriophage) and transferred to another organism of the same species. This is a relatively ineffective method of transfer, but is clinically important in the transfer of resistance genes between strains of staphylococci and streptococci.

Sulphonamides

Sulfadiazine is well absorbed following oral administration. Sulphonamides were used to treat 'simple' urinary tract infections, but many *Escherichia coli*† strains are resistant and much less toxic drugs are now available. Sulfadiazine in combination with pyrimethamine is used in infections of *Toxoplasma gondii* (toxoplasmosis).

Adverse effects

The most common side-effects are allergic reactions and include skin rashes (morbilliform or urticarial), sometimes with a fever. Much less common are more serious reactions, e.g. the Stevens–Johnson syndrome, which is a form of erythema multiforme with a high mortality rate. Various blood dyscrasias may occur, rarely, including agranulocytosis, aplastic anaemia and haemolytic anaemia (especially in patients with glucose-6-phosphodehydrogenase deficiency).

Trimethoprim is well absorbed orally and is effective in most patients with simple lower urinary tract infections. It is sometimes used for respiratory tract infections, but it has relatively poor activity against *Streptococcus pneumoniae* and *Streptococcus pyogenes*.

Co-trimoxazole (**trimethoprim** combined with **sulfamethoxazole**). Because the side-effects of co-trimoxazole are mainly the same as those of the sulphonamides, its use is now largely restricted to treating patients with *Pneumocystis jiroveci* pneumonia, *nocardiasis* and *toxoplasmosis*.

Quinolones

Nalidixic acid was the first quinolone found to have antibacterial activity, but it does not achieve systemic antibacterial levels and has been used only for urinary tract infections. **Ciprofloxacin** has a 6-fluoro substituent that confers greatly enhanced antibacterial potency against both Gram-positive and especially Gram-negative organisms, including *E. coli*, *Pseudomonas aeruginosa*, *Salmonella* and *Campylobacter*. So far, resistance is uncommon. Ciprofloxacin is well absorbed orally and can be given intravenously. It is eliminated, largely unchanged, mainly by the kidneys. Side-effects are infrequent, but include nausea, vomiting, rashes, dizziness, headache and, rarely, tendon damage. Convulsions may occur because the quinolones are γ-aminobutyric acid (GABA) antagonists. **Norfloxacin** has no systemic activity. It is concentrated in the urine and is a second-line drug in urinary tract infections.

5-Nitroimidazoles

Metronidazole is well absorbed orally and can be given intravenously. It is active against most anaerobic bacteria, including *Bacteroides* species. Metronidazole is the drug of choice in certain protozoal infections, i.e. *Entamoeba histolytica*, *Giardia lamblia*, and *Trichomonas vaginalis* (Chapter 43). Side-effects include gastrointestinal disturbances. **Tinidazole** has similar actions to metronidazole, but has a longer duration of action. It is useful in giardiasis where the high doses of metronidazole may be poorly tolerated.

---

† *Escherichia coli* is a Gram-negative rod and is the most common cause of urinary tract infections.

38 Antibacterial drugs that inhibit cell wall synthesis: penicillins, cephalosporins and vancomycin

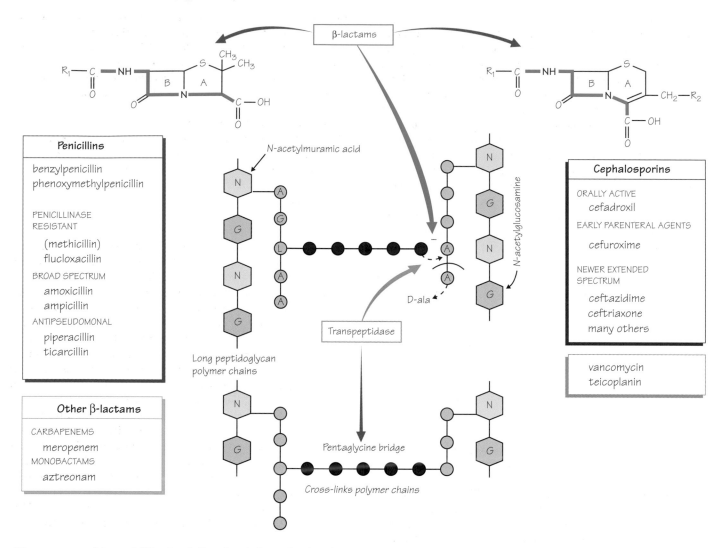

The structures of the penicillins (top left) and cephalosporins (top right) share the common feature of a β-lactam ring (B), the integrity of which is essential for antimicrobial activity. Modification of groups R_1 and R_2 has resulted in many semisynthetic antibiotics, some of which are acid resistant (and orally active), have a wide spectrum of antimicrobial activity, or are resistant to bacterial β-lactamases. Other β-lactams have been developed that are resistant to β-lactamases (bottom left). The penicillins (left) are the most important antibiotics*. The β-lactam antibiotics are bactericidal. They produce their antimicrobial action by preventing the cross-linkage between the linear peptidoglycan polymer chains that make up the bacterial cell wall, e.g. by a pentaglycine bridge (●). This action is because a part of their structure (━) resembles the D-alanyl-D-alanine of the peptide chains of the bacterial cell wall.

Benzylpenicillin was the first of the penicillins and remains important, but it is largely destroyed by gastric acid and must be given by injection. **Phenoxymethylpenicillin** has a similar antimicrobial spectrum, but is active orally. Many bacteria (including most staphylococci) are resistant to benzylpenicillin because they produce enzymes (β-lactamases, penicillinase) that open the β-lactam ring. The genetic control of β-lactamases often resides in transmissible plasmids (Chapter 37). Some penicillins, e.g. **flucloxacillin**, are effective against β-lactamase-producing staphylococci. Gram-negative, but not Gram-positive, bacteria possess an outer phospholipid membrane that may confer penicillin resistance by hindering access of the drugs to the cell wall. The **broad-spectrum** penicillins, such as **amoxicillin** and **ampicillin**, are more hydrophilic than benzylpenicillin and are active against some Gram-negative bacteria because they can pass through pores in the outer phospholipid membrane. Penicillinase-producing organisms are resistant to amoxicillin and ampicillin. The **antipseudomonal penicillins** (bottom left) are used mainly for the treatment of serious infections caused by *Pseudomonas aeruginosa*.†

* Antibiotics are chemotherapeutic agents made by living microorganisms rather than by chemical synthesis.

† *Pseudomonas aeruginosa* is a Gram-negative bacillus resistant to many antibiotics. It can cause serious opportunistic infections including pneumonia and septicaemia.

Penicillins have a very low toxicity, but high concentrations (renal failure, intrathecal administration) may produce encephalopathy, which can be fatal. **Hypersensitivity** is the most important side-effect of the penicillins, which may cause rashes and, rarely, **anaphylactic reactions** that are fatal in about 10% of cases.

Penicillins

Benzylpenicillin is still a useful antibiotic, but it has a 'narrow spectrum' of activity, mainly against Gram-positive organisms. Benzylpenicillin is effective for treating pneumococcal, streptococcal, meningococcal and leptospiral infections. It is also valuable for the prophylaxis of clostridial gas gangrene. Most *Staphylococcus aureus*‡ strains now produce penicillinase. Benzylpenicillin is acid labile and is therefore poorly absorbed orally. It is given by intramuscular injection, but large doses are painful and are given intravenously. Penicillin diffuses widely through the body tissues, but penetration into the brain is poor, except when the meninges are inflamed. Following intramuscular injection, peak plasma levels occur after 15–30 min and the drug is rapidly excreted (largely unchanged) by the kidneys. The elimination half-life ($t_{1/2}$) is normally 30 min, but is prolonged to about 10 h in anuria. The renal tubular secretion of penicillin can be inhibited by organic acids such as **probenecid**, and this results in higher and more prolonged plasma concentrations.

Phenoxymethylpenicillin has the same spectrum as benzylpenicillin, but is less active. It is acid stable and is given orally. However, its absorption is variable and it is only useful for very sensitive organisms, where a rapid action is unnecessary (streptococcal tonsillitis). Phenoxymethylpenicillin is useful in the prophylaxis of rheumatic fever.

Penicillinase-resistant penicillins: flucloxacillin

Flucloxacillin is indicated in infections caused by penicillinase-producing penicillin-resistant staphylococci. It is a semisynthetic penicillin and is resistant to penicillinase because an isoxazolyl group at R_1 sterically hinders access of the enzyme to the β-lactam ring. Flucloxacillin is less effective than benzylpenicillin and should only be used in infections caused by penicillinase-producing staphylococci (which includes most hospital-acquired staphylococcal infections). Flucloxacillin is well absorbed orally but, in severe infections, it should be given by injection and not be used alone. Epidemic strains of *Staphylococcus aureus* resistant to methicillin (MRSA), flucloxacillin and other antibiotics are an increasing problem, especially in hospitals. Such infections may be sensitive to intravenous vancomycin or teicoplanin.

Broad-spectrum penicillins

Ampicillin and **amoxicillin** are active against non-β-lactamase-producing Gram-positive bacteria, and, because they diffuse into Gram-negative bacteria more readily than benzylpenicillin, they are also active against many strains of *Escherichia coli*, *Haemophilis influenzae* and *Salmonella*. For oral administration, amoxicillin is the drug of choice, because it is better absorbed than ampicillin, which should be given parenterally. Amoxicillin and ampicillin are inactivated by penicillinase-producing bacteria. Organisms that are resistant to amoxicillin include most *Staphylococcus aureus*, 50% of

‡ *Staphylococcus aureus* is a Gram-positive coccus. It is a common cause of infections, including boils, wound infections, pneumonia, endocarditis and septicaemia.

Escherichia coli strains and up to 15% of *Haemophilis influenzae* strains. Many bacterial β-lactamases are inhibited by *clavulanic acid*, and a mixture of this inhibitor with **amoxicillin (co-amoxiclav)** results in the antibiotic being effective against penicillinase-producing organisms. Co-amoxiclav is indicated in respiratory and urinary tract infections, which are confirmed to be resistant to amoxicillin.

Antipseudomonal penicillins

Piperacillin and **ticarcillin** are given by injection for serious infections with Gram-negative bacteria, especially *Pseudomonas aeruginosa*. They can be combined with aminoglycosides for the initial treatment of serious infection (e.g. septicaemia, endocarditis) when the bacterial cause has not been identified.

Cephalosporins

The cephalosporin antibiotics are used for the treatment of meningitis, pneumonia and septicaemia. The cephalosporins have the same mechanism of action as, and similar pharmacology to, penicillin. They may produce allergic reactions, and cross-sensitivity to penicillin may occur. They are excreted mainly by the kidneys and their actions can be prolonged with probenecid. They all have a similar broad spectrum of antibacterial activity, although individual drugs have different activity against certain bacteria. **Cefadroxil** is administered orally and is used in urinary tract infections where the organisms are resistant to other antibiotics. **Cefuroxime** is given by injection, often as a prophylactic in surgery (usually with metronidazole to provide cover against anaerobes). Cefuroxime is resistant to inactivation by bacterial β-lactamases and is used in serious infections when other antibiotics are ineffective. **Ceftazidime** has an increased range of activity against Gram-negative bacteria, including *Pseudomonas aeruginosa*, but is less active than cefuroxime against Gram-positive organisms (e.g. *Staphylococcus aureus*). It reaches the central nervous system and is used in meningitis caused by Gram-negative organisms. **Ceftriaxone** has a longer half-life than other cephalosporins and only needs to be given once a day.

Other β-lactam antibiotics

Meropenem is a carbapenem (a structure similar to penicillin), but is highly resistant to β-lactamases. It has a wide spectrum of activity, but is inactive against some *Pseudomonas* strains and MRSA. It is given by intravenous injection.

Vancomycin

Vancomycin is a bactericidal antibiotic that is not absorbed orally. It acts by inhibiting peptidoglycan formation and is active against most Gram-positive organisms. Intravenous vancomycin is important for the treatment of patients with septicaemia or endocarditis caused by methicillin-resistant strains of *Staphylococcus aureus*. It is given orally for antibiotic-associated pseudomembranous colitis (a serious complication of antibiotic therapy caused by a superinfection of the bowel by *Clostridium difficile*, which produces a toxin that damages the colonic mucosa). An alternative is metronidazole (Chapter 37). Rarely, vancomycin may cause renal failure or hearing loss.

39 Antibacterial drugs that inhibit protein synthesis: aminoglycosides, tetracyclines, macrolides and chloramphenicol

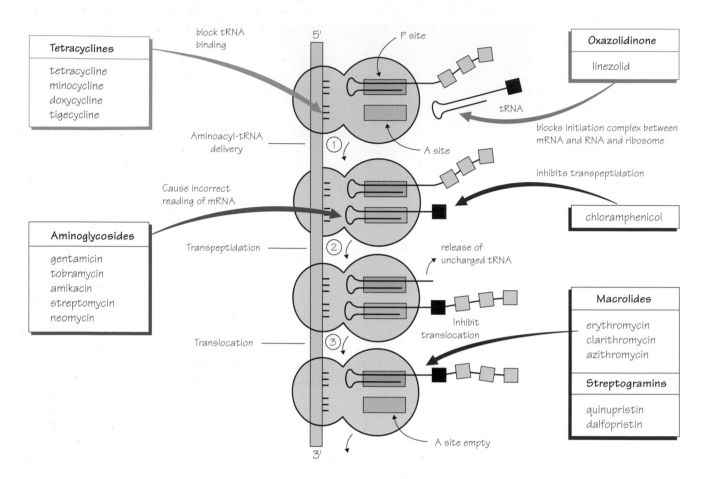

This group of antibiotics acts by inhibiting bacterial protein synthesis. They are selectively toxic because bacterial ribosomes (the sites of protein synthesis) consist of a 50S and a 30S subunit, whereas mammalian ribosomes have a 60S and a 40S subunit.

Proteins are built from amino acids, on ribosomes (⬭), which move along (1–2–3) strands of messenger ribonucleic acid (mRNA, ▯) so that successive codons (⊔⊔) pass through an acceptor (aminoacyl, A site, ▭) for specific transfer RNA (tRNA) molecules that bear the next amino acid (top right, ◼) required to elongate the peptide chain. The **tetracyclines** (top left) and **aminoglycosides** (bottom left) bind to the 30S subunit and inhibit binding of the aminoacyl-tRNA. In addition, the aminoglycosides cause *misreading* of mRNA, so that nonfunctional proteins are synthesized. The next step in peptide synthesis is transpeptidation (2), where the growing peptide chain (▭▭), attached to the P (peptidyl, ▭) site, is transferred to the amino acid (◼) attached to the aminoacyl-tRNA at the A site. **Chloramphenicol** (middle right) *inhibits peptidyl transferase* activity of the 50S ribosomal subunit. Following transpeptidation, the peptide chain is translocated from site A to P (3), so that the A site is ready to accept the next

aminoacyl-tRNA. The **macrolides** and **streptogramins** (bottom right) bind to the 50S subunit and *inhibit translocation*. The streptogramins, **quinupristin** and **dalfopristin**, are bactericidal drugs that are active against many Gram-positive bacteria. They are reserved for serious infections resistant to other drugs, e.g. methicillin-resistant *Staphylococcus aureus* (MRSA).

The **aminoglycosides**, such as **gentamicin**, must be given by injection. They are valuable drugs in the treatment of severe infections, but are likely to produce nephrotoxic and ototoxic effects. The **tetracyclines** are orally active, wide-spectrum antibiotics, but increasing bacterial resistance has reduced their usefulness. **Macrolides** (e.g. **erythromycin**) have a similar antibacterial spectrum to benzylpenicillin. Gram-positive bacteria are more sensitive than Gram-negative bacteria to erythromycin because they accumulate about 100 times more drug. **Chloramphenicol** is effective against a wide range of organisms, but serious side-effects (e.g. aplastic anaemia) restrict its use. **Linezolid** is a newer drug with a novel mechanism of action. It is currently active against MRSA and vancomycin-resistant enterococci. Adverse effects include marrow suppression and peripheral neuropathy.

Aminoglycosides

The **aminoglycosides** are not absorbed orally and must be given by injection. They are bactericidal and are active against many Gram-negative and some Gram-positive organisms. The aminoglycosides have a narrow therapeutic index and are all potentially toxic. They are excreted by the kidney, and renal impairment results in accumulation and a greater risk of toxic side-effects. The most important side-effects of the aminoglycosides are damage to the VIIIth cranial nerve (**ototoxicity**) and damage to the **kidneys**. These effects are dose related, and assays of blood aminoglycoside levels should be carried out regularly on all patients receiving aminoglycosides. Aminoglycosides may impair neuromuscular transmission and are therefore contraindicated in patients with myasthenia gravis.

Resistance to aminoglycosides arises from several mechanisms, the most important being the production of enzymes (plasmid-controlled) that inactivate the drug by acetylation, phosphorylation or adenylation. Other mechanisms are the alterations of the envelope to prevent drug access and alteration of the binding site on the 30S subunit so that the drug does not bind (streptomycin only).

Gentamicin is the most important aminoglycoside, its main use being in the 'empirical' treatment of acute life-threatening Gram-negative infections (e.g. *Pseudomonas aeruginosa*) in hospitals, until antibiotic sensitivities are known. Gentamicin may have a synergistic antimicrobial action with penicillin and vancomycin, and combinations with one of these agents are used in the treatment of streptococcal endocarditis. **Amikacin** is less affected by aminoglycoside-inactivating enzymes and is used in serious Gram-negative infections that are gentamicin resistant. **Neomycin** is too toxic for parenteral use. It is used topically in skin infections, and orally to sterilize the bowel prior to surgery.

Streptomycin is active against *Mycobacterium tuberculosis*. However, because it causes dose-related **ototoxicity**, especially with prolonged or intensive therapy, it has been largely replaced by **rifampicin** (Chapter 37). Resistance rapidly develops to rifampicin alone and, in the **treatment of tuberculosis**, it is combined with **isoniazid**, **ethambutol** and **pyrazinamide** for the first 2 months of treatment. Then treatment is continued for another 4 months, usually with rifampicin and isoniazid. Ethambutol, isoniazid and pyrazinamide are active only against *M. tuberculosis*, but their mechanisms of action are unknown.

Macrolides

Macrolides* are usually given orally, but **erythromycin** and **clarithromycin** can be given intravenously if necessary. They have a similar antimicrobial spectrum to benzylpenicillin (i.e. narrow spectrum, mainly active against Gram-positive organisms) and can be used as an alternative drug in penicillin-sensitive patients, especially in infections caused by streptococci, staphylococci, pneumococci and clostridia. However, they are ineffective in meningitis because they do not penetrate the central nervous system adequately. Unlike penicillin, the macrolides are effective against several unusual organisms and are specifically indicated in *Mycoplasma pneumoniae* and Legionnaires' disease. Resistance to macrolides may occur because of plasmid-controlled alteration of their receptor on the 50S subunit of the bacterial ribosomes (reducing binding).

Erythromycin is metabolized by the liver, and dosage reduction in renal failure is unnecessary unless there is severe failure. The macrolides are very safe drugs. Erythromycin in high doses may cause nausea and vomiting, but these effects are less common with azithromycin and clarithromycin. Azithromycin has a very long half-life (40–60 h) and a single dose is as effective in the treatment of chlamydial non-specific urethritis as tetracycline administered for 7 days. The macrolides inhibit cytochrome P450 and cause accumulation of warfarin.

Tetracyclines

Tetracyclines are usually given orally, but may be given by injection. Absorption from the gut is variable and is reduced by calcium ions (milk), magnesium ions (e.g. antacids), food and iron preparations. Tetracyclines are broad-spectrum antibiotics, but there are more suitable agents for most infections. However, they are the drugs of choice for treating some infections caused by intracellular organisms, because they penetrate macrophages well, e.g. *Chlamydia* (non-specific urethritis, trachoma, psittacosis), rickettsia (Q-fever) and *Borrelia burgdorferi* (Lyme disease). Organisms sensitive to tetracyclines accumulate the drug partly by passive diffusion and partly by active transport. Resistant organisms produce an efflux pump and do not accumulate the antibiotic. Tetracyclines bind to calcium in growing bones and teeth. This causes discoloration of the teeth in the young, and tetracyclines should be avoided in children up to 8 years of age and in pregnant or lactating women. Diarrhoea and nausea may occur. Overgrowth with *Candida albicans* in the mouth or bowel sometimes leads to thrush. In general, the properties of the tetracyclines are similar. One exception is **tigecycline**, a newer glycylcycline antibacterial structually similar to minocycline. Its 9-glycylamide structure seems to confer protection from the two commonest resistance mechanisms, i.e. efflux pumps and ribosomal alteration. Tigecycline is given by intravenous infusion and is active against a wide range of pathogens including MRSA and vancomycin-resistant enterococci. It is effective for intra-abdominal, skin, and soft-tissue infections.

Chloramphenicol

Chloramphenicol is given orally or by intravenous injection. It is effective against a wide range of organisms. Serious adverse effects, which include bone marrow aplasia (incidence about 1 in 40 000 – usually fatal), reversible (dose-related) suppression of red and white blood cells, and peripheral and optic neuritis, restrict its use for systemic infections. Chloramphenicol is now reserved for the treatment of typhoid fever and *Haemophilus influenzae* meningitis, but a wide-spectrum cephalosporin is usually preferred. Chloramphenicol is widely used topically to treat bacterial conjunctivitis. It is metabolized mainly in the liver and penetrates widely, including the brain.

Streptogramins

Quinupristin and **dalfopristin** are cyclic peptides and act in a similar way to the macrolides. They are given in combination because individually they are less effective. Quinupristin/dalfopristin are given by intravenous infusion and are active against many Gram-positive organisms. Adverse effects include nausea, vomiting, diarrhoea, myalgia and arthralgia.

* Macrolide: a many-membered lactone ring to which one or more deoxy sugars are attached.

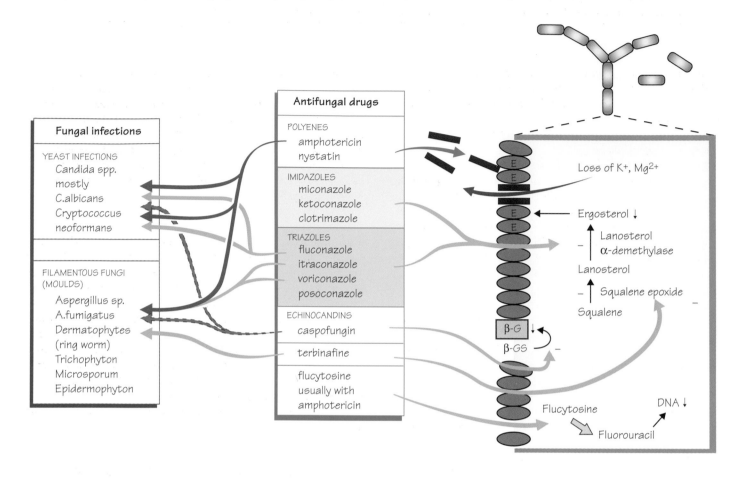

Fungal infections (mycoses) (left) result in a wide range of diseases. Some superficial infections are relatively trivial, e.g. athlete's foot, but invasive systemic infections, which occur mostly in immunocompromised patients (AIDS patients, corticosteroids, anticancer and immunosuppresive drugs), are often life-threatening and require intensive therapy. Pathogenic fungi do not produce toxins, but in the host they often produce hypersensitivity reactions. In systemic mycoses the typical tissue reaction is chronic granuloma formation with varying degrees of necrosis and abscess formation. Invasive mycoses in immunocompromised patients have a high mortality rate (e.g. 30–60% in *Candida albicans* infections).

For many years, the first-line drug in severe and potentially fatal systemic mycoses has been **amphotericin** (top, centre), an effective but highly toxic drug. Amphotericin is a polyene antibiotic that binds (right, ■) to ergosterol (E) in the fungal cell membrane and forms channels through which essential fungal cell constituents (e.g. potassium) are lost (◄─). The drug has a relatively selective action on fungal cells because, in human cells, the major sterol is cholesterol rather than ergosterol. Amphotericin is not absorbed orally and is given by intravenous infusion to treat systemic fungal infections. Lipid formulations are much less toxic and allow higher doses to be administered. **Nystatin** has a similar structure to amphotericin but is not absorbed from mucous membranes and its use is limited to *Candida albicans* infections of the skin and mucous membranes. **Flucytosine** (bottom, centre) is much less toxic than amphotericin, but its use is limited because it has a narrow spectrum and resistance can develop rapidly during therapy. Flucytosine is converted in fungal cells, but not in human cells, into fluorouracil (⟐), which inhibits fungal DNA synthesis (Chapter 44). Flucytosine is used with amphotericin to produce a synergistic action.

The **imidazoles** (centre, ▢) are broad-spectrum antifungal drugs that are widely used topically. They inhibit cytochrome lanosterol-α-demethylase, an enzyme that converts lanosterol to ergosterol. This causes lanosterol to accumulate and leads to perturbation of the fungal cell membrane and fungistasis. The **triazoles** (centre, ▢) are structurally similar to the imidazoles, but with a wider range of antifungal activity. They have a lower incidence of adverse effects because they are much more specific inhibitors of lanosterol α-demethylase (right).

Confirmed dermatophyte infections of the nails or skin are treated with **terbinafine**, a drug that inhibits squalene epoxide (centre, right) and leads to toxic levels of squalene accumulating in the fungal cells (centre, right). **Griseofulvin** has been used for some dermatophyte infections, particularly scalp ringworm. It is rarely used now, having been replaced by more effective drugs.

The **echinocandins**, e.g. **caspofungin**, are a new class of antifungal drugs. They are large lipopeptide molecules. Caspofungin has a fatty acid side chain that is thought to intercalate with the phospholipid bilayer of the cell membrane. Echinocandins act by inhibiting the synthetic cell wall enzyme complex β-(1,3)-D-glucan synthase (β-GS, right). This prevents the synthesis of β-(1,3)-glucan, an essential polysaccharide component of the rigid fungal cell wall, and causes osmotic lysis of the fungal cells.

Fungal infections

There are three main groups of fungi that cause disease in humans:

1 Moulds (filamentous fungi) grow as long filaments that intertwine to form a mycelium. Examples are the *dermatophytes*, so called because of their ability to digest keratin, which cause infections of the skin, nails and hair, and *Aspergillus fumigatus*, which may cause pulmonary or disseminated aspergillosis.

2 True yeasts are unicellular round or oval fungi, e.g. *Cryptococcus neoformans*, which may cause cryptococcal meningitis or pulmonary infections, usually only in immunocompromised patients.

3 Yeast-like fungi are similar to yeasts, but may also form long, non-branching filaments. An important example is *Candida albicans*, which is a common commensal organism in the gut, mouth and vagina. It causes a wide range of diseases, including oral thrush, vaginitis, endocarditis and septicaemia (often fatal).

Polyenes

Amphotericin is a wide-spectrum antifungal drug used to treat potentially fatal systemic infections caused by *Aspergillus*, *Candida* or *Cryptococcus*. It is poorly absorbed orally and is given by intravenous infusion, or intrathecally when the central nervous system is involved. Adverse effects are very common and most patients develop fever, chills and nausea. Long-term therapy almost inevitably causes renal damage, which is reversible only if detected early. Amphotericin formulated in liposomes is less toxic and increasingly used. **Nystatin** is too toxic for parenteral use. It is mainly used for *Candida albicans* infections of the skin (as a cream or ointment) and mucous membranes (as tablets sucked in the mouth, vaginal pessaries). Oropharyngeal candidiasis (thrush) is one of the most common features of AIDS and is sometimes a sequel to the use of broad-spectrum antibiotics, anticancer drugs or corticosteroids.

Flucytosine

Flucytosine is given by intravenous infusion and is used mainly to treat systemic candidiasis or cryptococcal infections. As resistance often develops rapidly, flucytosine is often given in combination with amphotericin. The drugs act synergistically and the combination is effective in cryptococcal meningitis.

Imidazoles

Imidazoles are wide-spectrum antifungal drugs to which resistance rarely develops. Except for ketoconazole, the imidazoles are poorly absorbed orally. **Clotrimazole**, **econazole** and **miconazole** are widely used topically in the treatment of dermatophyte and *Candida albicans* infections. **Ketoconazole** is well absorbed orally, and has been used in the treatment of local and systemic mycoses. The adverse effects of ketoconazole include hepatic necrosis and adrenal suppression, and it has been superseded by fluconazole and itraconazole for the treatment of systemic mycoses.

Triazoles

Fluconazole may be given orally or intravenously. It is widely distributed and crosses the blood–brain barrier. It is active against *Candida* and *Cryptococcus* but not against filamentous fungi (i.e. *Aspergillus*). Fluconazole is used orally to treat oropharyngeal and oesophageal candidiasis, and intravenously to treat systemic candidiasis and cryptococcal infections, including cryptococcal meningitis. Fluconazole is well tolerated although it may cause liver enzyme abnormalities. It does, however, undergo significant drug interactions, and high doses may increase the actions of phenytoin, ciclosporin, zidovudine and warfarin.

Itraconazole is absorbed orally and, unlike the imidazoles and fluconazole, is active against *Aspergillus*.

Voriconazole is a newer broad-spectrum drug used for life-threatening infections.

Echinocandins

The echinocandins are poorly absorbed when given orally and are administered by intravenous infusion. **Caspofungin** is used in invasive aspergillosis and candidiasis unresponsive to amphotericin or itraconazole. The low toxicity of the echinocandins compared with amphotericin is leading to their increased use in the treatment of these infections. Adverse effects of caspofungin include headache, nausea and hypokalaemia.

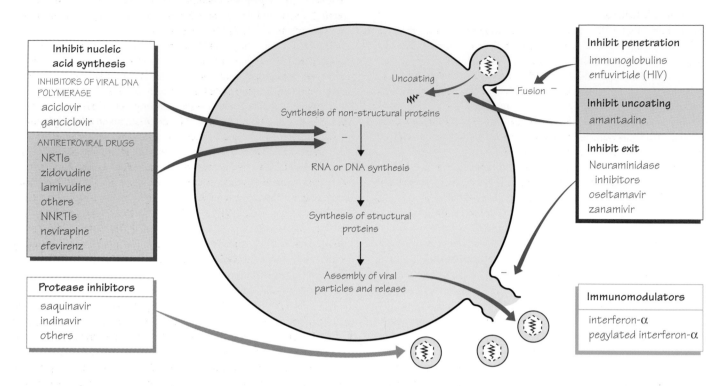

Inhibit nucleic acid synthesis

INHIBITORS OF VIRAL DNA POLYMERASE
aciclovir
ganciclovir

ANTIRETROVIRAL DRUGS
NRTIs
zidovudine
lamivudine
others
NNRTIs
nevirapine
efevirenz

Protease inhibitors
saquinavir
indinavir
others

Inhibit penetration
immunoglobulins
enfuvirtide (HIV)

Inhibit uncoating
amantadine

Inhibit exit
Neuraminidase
  inhibitors
oseltamivir
zanamivir

Immunomodulators
interferon-α
pegylated interferon-α

Uncoating
Fusion
Synthesis of non-structural proteins
RNA or DNA synthesis
Synthesis of structural proteins
Assembly of viral particles and release

Viruses are intracellular parasites that lack independent metabolism and can replicate only within living host cells. Because their replication cycle is so intimately connected with the metabolic processes of the host cell, it has proved extremely difficult to produce drugs that are selectively toxic to viruses. For this reason, vaccines have been the main method for controlling viral infections (e.g. poliomyelitis, rabies, yellow fever, measles, mumps, rubella). However, the HIV-1 pandemic stimulated a search for new antiviral drugs, and in the last 15 years or so many effective antiviral drugs have been produced. These have transformed the treatment of several diseases, notably those caused by HIV-1 and herpes virus infections.

Viral replication involves several steps (figure, centre). The first stage involves fusion of the virus with the host cell, followed by entry and uncoating of the virus. **Enfuvirtide** (used in AIDs) and **immunoglobulins** (top right) inhibit penetration of the cell by the virus, whilst **amantadine** (right, shaded) inhibits the uncoating of influenza-virus A once it has entered the cell. The neuraminidase inhibitors (centre, right), e.g. **oseltamivir**, prevent the exit of new virions from the host cell.

Many antiviral drugs (left) interfere with viral (and often human) nucleic acid synthesis. Drugs that act by inhibiting viral DNA polymerase, e.g. **aciclovir** (top, left), are more selectively antiviral because they are inactive until phosphorylated by enzymes that are preferentially synthesized by the virus. Aciclovir is used in the treatment of herpes virus infections.

Antiretroviral drugs (middle left, shaded) are used to suppress the replication of human immunodeficiency virus (HIV) in patients with AIDS. Resistance to single drugs develops rapidly and this unfortunate fact led to the introduction of highly active antiretroviral treatments (**HAART**). HAART involves the use of various drug combinations, e.g. two nucleoside reverse transcriptase inhibitors (**NRTIs**) with either a non-nucleoside reverse transcriptase inhibitor (**NNRTI**) or a **protease inhibitor** (bottom, left). HAART does not eradicate HIV infection but has led to a dramatic reduction in AIDS-associated morbidity and mortality and has raised the hope that HIV-1 infection can be transformed into a treatable chronic disease. However, HAART is associated with many adverse effects, and although these are outweighed by the benefits in patients with clinical signs of immunodeficiency or low CD4 cell numbers, their use in asymptomatic patients is more controversial. One strategy to try to reduce long-term drug toxicity has been the introduction of drug 'holidays', during which the body's own immune system could keep the virus in check. However, a recent trial showed that interruption of treatment was associated with increased morbidity and mortality. Thus, at present, most experts strongly discourage treatment interruption, except in cases of treatment intolerance.

The **interferons** (bottom, right) are drugs that modulate the host immune system. Recombinant interferon alfa is given by injection in the treatment of chronic persistent hepatitis B and in combination with ribavirin in chronic hepatitis C.

Drugs that prevent the virus entering or leaving the host cells

Immunoglobulins

Human immunoglobulin contains specific antibodies against superficial antigens of viruses and can interfere with their entry into host cells. Normal immunoglobulin injections are used to give temporary protection against hepatitis A, measles and rubella. **Enfuvirtide** is the first antiretroviral drug to act by preventing the entry of HIV-1 virus into host cells. It is a synthetic peptide that mimics amino acids 127–162 of HIV-1 gp41, which is a key domain in membrane fusion. It is given by subcutaneous injection, as an additional drug, in patients who are failing to respond to other antiretroviral agents.

Palivizumab is a monoclonal antibody that binds to a glycoprotein on the suface of respiratory syncytial virus (RSV) and prevents attachment to host cells (cf. immunoglobulins). It is given monthly by intramuscular injection to infants at high risk of RSV infections.

Amantadine

Amantadine is an older drug that is now rarely used. It interferes with the replication of influenza virus A by inhibiting the transmembrane M2 protein that is essential for uncoating the virus. It has a narrow spectrum and influenza vaccine is usually preferable.

Neuraminidase inhibitors

Neuraminidase and haemagglutin are antigenic proteins expressed as spikes on the envelope of influenza virus. The virus enters the host cell by endocytosis. Hydrogen ions then enter the endosome though the M2 ion channel causing disassembly of the virus and leading to replication of the RNA virus. The new virions exit the host cell by budding from the cell membrane, a process that requires *neuraminidase* to sever the bonds linking the viral coat to the host sialic acid. The **neuraminidase inhibitors**, **zanamivir** and **oseltamivir**, reduce the symptoms of influenza by about 1 day and are most effective if started within a few hours of the onset of symptoms. Zanamivir is given by inhalation but oseltamivir (*Tamiflu*) is given orally and can be used for prophylaxis. Whether these drugs would be effective in an avian flu epidemic is unknown.

Drugs that inhibit nucleic acid synthesis

Aciclovir (acyclovir, acycloguanosine). The herpes viruses, e.g. *herpes simplex virus* (HSV) and *varicella zoster virus* (VZV), contain a thymidine kinase that converts aciclovir to a monophosphate. The monophosphate is subsequently phosphorylated by host cell enzymes to acycloguanosine triphosphate, which inhibits viral DNA polymerase and viral DNA synthesis. Aciclovir is selectively toxic because the thymidine kinase of uninfected host cells activates only a little of the drug, and the DNA polymerase of herpes virus has a much higher affinity than the cellular DNA polymerase for the activated drug. Aciclovir is active against herpes viruses, but does not eradicate them. It is effective topically, orally and parenterally, and the appropriate route depends on the site and severity of the infection. Aciclovir is widely used in the treatment of HSV genital infections, and high oral doses are effective in treating severe shingles, a painful condition caused by reactivation of a previous infection with VZV (i.e. chickenpox).

Ganciclovir must be given intravenously and, because of its toxicity (neutropenia), it is used only to treat severe cytomegalovirus (CMV) infections in immunocompromised patients. CMV is resistant to aciclovir because it does not code for thymidine kinase.

Zidovudine inhibits the reverse transcriptase of HIV and is used orally in the treatment of AIDS. The drug is activated by triple phosphorylation and then binds to reverse transcriptase, for which it has 100 times the affinity that it has for cellular DNA polymerases. The drug is incorporated into the DNA chain and, because it lacks a 3′-hydroxyl, another nucleotide cannot form a 3′–5′ phosphodiester bond and so the DNA chain is terminated. Some patients cannot tolerate the severe side-effects, which include anaemia, neutropenia, myalgia, nausea and headaches. Other NRTIs include **stavudine**, **didanosine** and **zalcitabine**. Newer NNRTIs that act by denaturing reverse transcriptase include **nevirapine** and **efavirenz**.

Protease inhibitors

In HIV, mRNAs are translated into inert polyproteins. These are then converted into essential mature proteins (e.g. reverse transcriptase) by a virus-specific protease. Inhibitors of 'HIV protease' prevent the maturation of virions resulting in the production of non-infectious particles. They are used in combination with other drugs and include **saquinavir** and **ritonavir**. Adverse effects include nausea, vomiting, diabetes and lipodystrophy.

Immunomodulators

Interferons (**IFNs**) are protective glycoproteins that are synthesized in the body in response to virus infection. They are classified as α, β or γ. Interferons have a wide spectrum of activity. They prevent viral replication by binding to specific ganglioside receptors on the host cells and induce the production of enzymes that inhibit the translation of viral mRNA into viral proteins.

IFN-α is effective in a number of conditions including chronic myelogenous leukaemia, Kaposi's sarcoma and chronic hepatitis B and C. IFNs conjugated with polyethylene glycol (**pegylated IFNs**) have a longer action and are more effective. Hepatitis B (HBV) is treated with pegylated IFN-α but the response rate is less than 50% and relapse is frequent. **Lamivudine** has activity against HBV but resistant strains may develop. Some newer drugs, e.g. **adefovir**, are effective in lamivudine-resistant infections. Antiviral suppression of HBV for 2–5 years reverses hepatic fibrosis and prevents cirrhosis. Hepatitis C (HCV) is treated with **pegylated IFN-α** and **ribavirin**, and this combination successfully clears the virus in over 50% of patients. Adverse effects are common and include lethargy, anorexia, depression and an influenza-like syndrome.

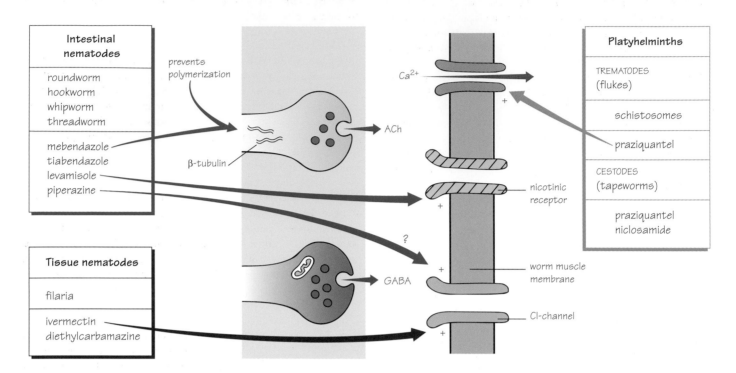

Parasitism is a relationship in which one biological species lives in a dependent association with another. Although microorganisms such as bacteria may be considered to be in such a relationship, only the **protozoa** and **helminths** are generally referred to as parasites. They typically are eukaryotic and have complex life cycles. Only a few parasitic diseases are common in Great Britain (e.g. threadworms, giardiasis; Chapter 43), but, in tropical and subtropical areas, where abundant water and high temperatures provide an optimal environment for the larvae and intermediate vector hosts (e.g. mosquitoes), parasitic diseases are common and widespread. Overcrowding, malnutrition and lack of sanitation facilitate the spread of disease, and more than half the world's population is thought to be infected with parasites. Drugs play an important part in the treatment and control of parasitic diseases, but other methods, e.g. vector control by insecticides and land drainage, are also important.

The **helminths** are worms that are round (**nematodes**, left) or flat (**platyhelminths**, right). The flatworms are divided into tapeworms (**cestodes**, bottom right) and flukes (**trematodes**, top right). The *nervous system* of helminths has important differences from that of vertebrates, and these differences form the basis of the selective toxicity of most drugs used to treat infections with worms (**anthelmintics**).

Nematode muscles have both excitatory and inhibitory neuromuscular junctions, the transmitters being acetylcholine (ganglion-type nicotinic receptors) and γ-aminobutyric acid (GABA), respectively. **Levamisole** (centre left) stimulates the nicotinic receptors at the neuromuscular junction and causes a spastic paralysis that results in the worms being expelled. **Ivermectin** (bottom left), a more recent drug that is effective against most nematodes, may enhance GABA-mediated inhibition at the neuromuscular junction, whereas **piperazine** (centre left) may act as a GABA agonist. Both drugs cause flaccid paralysis of the worms. GABAergic drugs are ineffective against trematodes and cestodes because they do not have peripheral GABAergic nerves. **Praziquantel** (right), a highly effective agent, induces muscular contraction and spastic paralysis in these parasites by increasing calcium fluxes. Some anthelmintics have quite well-characterized biochemical actions. In particular, the benzimidazole derivatives, e.g. **mebendazole** (centre left), bind to β-tubulin in nematode cells with a much greater affinity than they do to human tubulin, and block the transport of secretory granules and other organelles. The mechanism of action of some anthelmintics is unknown, e.g. **diethylcarbamazine**, a drug used in the treatment of lymphatic filariasis. It is possible that diethylcarbamazine alters the parasite so that it becomes susceptible to the host immune system.

Nematodes (roundworms)

Ascaris lumbricoides (common roundworm) infects the gut lumen in about 25% of the world's population. The worms, which are between 10 and 30 cm in length, are common in the subtropics, especially in areas where sanitation is poor. Treatment is with oral **mebendazole** or **levamisole**. **Piperazine** is also effective, but may cause vomiting and diarrhoea.

Hookworm is infection of the gut with either *Ancylostoma duodenale* or *Necator americanus*. These small worms (about 1 cm in length) grip the mucosa and take a little blood from the host each day. Hookworm is a common cause of iron-deficiency anaemia in tropical and subtropical countries. **Mebendazole** is effective.

Strongyloides infects the gut, but many people infected with these small worms (2 mm in length) are asymptomatic. Treatment is with **tiabendazole**, **albendazole** or **ivermectin**.

Threadworms (pinworm). Infection with *Enterobius vermicularis* (about 1 cm in length) is very common, especially in children. Pruritus ani is the main symptom. Female worms deposit eggs on the perianal skin and this causes irritation. The larvae are often reingested via the fingers, and this maintains a cycle of autoinfection. The whole family is usually treated with **mebendazole**.

Whipworms. *Trichuris trichiura* causes infection of the gut lumen, often together with *Ascaris* and hookworms. Light asymptomatic infection is common. **Mebendazole** is effective.

Filarial infections. Both the adult and larval (microfilariae) forms of the filariae occur in humans. Transmission is by the bite of blood-sucking insects. The adult worms are very long-lived, and the shedding of microfilariae lasts for many years. The severity of the disease depends on the adult worm burden of the host.

Lymphatic filariasis is infection, usually with *Wuchereria bancrofti*, *Brugia malayi* or *B. timori*, transmitted by the bite of mosquito vectors. Adult worms living in the lymphatic vessels cause pathological changes that may result in obstructive lymphoedema. About 90 million people are infected, two-thirds of them living in China, India and Indonesia.

Onchocerciasis is infection with *Onchocerca volvulus* and occurs mainly in tropical Africa and Central America. Transmission is by blackflies of the genus *Simulium*. Most human infections are acquired near rivers because these are required by the blackfly to breed. Death of the microfilariae in the skin causes chronic pruritus, and in the cornea eventually causes scarring and blindness (river blindness).

Diethylcarbamazine and ivermectin are used in filarial infections. Onchocerciasis was, for many years, treated with **diethylcarbamazine**, which kills microfilariae (by an unknown mechanism) but not adult worms. Unfortunately, killing the microfilariae exacerbates the disease, often with severe reactions when there are lesions in the eyes. **Ivermectin** causes much less exacerbation of the disease and is now the treatment of choice.

Toxocariasis is caused by infection with larval forms of *Toxocara canis* or *T. cati*. Eggs shed in the faeces of dogs and cats are ingested (most often by children) and release larvae, which become dis-seminated to many organs including the eye. Dead worms evoke granuloma formation and may cause blindness. Treatment is with **diethylcarbamazine**, which kills migrating worms, but cannot affect fibrosing lesions already present.

Trematodes (flukes)

Schistosomiasis (bilharziasis) is infection with flukes of the genus *Schistosoma*; these flukes affect the bladder and urinary tract (*S. haematobium*) or intestine (*S. mansoni*, *S. japonicum*). The secondary host is an aquatic snail that releases cercariae into the water. Children are infected early in life by playing in infected water. Treatment is with **praziquantel**, which is effective in all fluke infections (except the liver fluke *Fasciola hepatica*).

Cestodes (tapeworms)

Taenia saginata and *Taenia solium* infections occur after eating undercooked infected beef and pork, respectively. The scolex evaginates from the ingested cysticercus (larval stage) and fixes to the gut wall. Then, self-fertile proglottids develop. The worm may be 5–10 m in length, but often causes no symptoms. Fish tapeworm (*Diphyllobothrium latum*) infection is acquired by eating infected uncooked fish. **Praziquantel** is effective in tapeworm infections.

Anthelmintics

Mebendazole, **tiabendazole** and **albendazole** are benzimidazoles given orally. They have a wide range of action, especially against intestinal nematodes. Mebendazole and albendazole have few side-effects, probably because they have low systemic bioavailability.

Levamisole is very effective in roundworm infections. It is given orally and paralyses the worms, which are then expelled in the faeces. Levamisole very rarely causes nausea or vomiting.

Ivermectin binds to invertebrate GABA receptors with an affinity about 100 times greater than that for vertebrate receptors, and may paralyse the worms by increasing GABA-mediated inhibition. However, more recent studies suggest that ivermectin activates a glutamate-gated chloride channel found only in invertebrates. Cestodes and trematodes lack high-affinity binding sites for ivermectin and so the drug is ineffective against these helminths. Ivermectin is active against the microfilariae of *O. volvulus*, but not the adult worm. It is also highly effective against ascariasis, enterobiasis, trichuriasis and strongyloidiasis. Ivermectin is given orally and has few side-effects. A single dose of the drug, given every 6–12 months, controls, but does not cure, onchocerciasis.

Praziquantel is given orally and has no serious unwanted effects. It is highly effective against many trematodes and cestodes (but not nematodes). The drug is taken up by susceptible helminths and binds to β-subunit of the schistosome voltage-gated Ca^{2+} channels. This induces an influx of Ca^{2+} ions and results in spastic paralysis and detachment of the worms. Perhaps more importantly, praziquantel damages the tegmentum, causing activation of host defence mechanisms and destruction of the helminths.

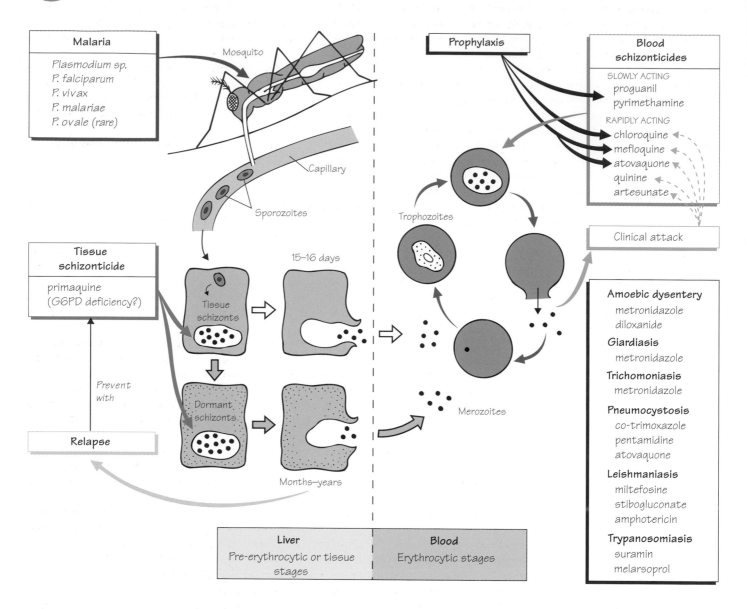

Malaria is the most serious protozoal disease, accounting for more than 1 million deaths a year; although it is not endemic in Europe or North America, travellers to malarial areas risk infection. This risk can be greatly reduced by taking prophylactic drugs (prophylaxis, top right), but multidrug-resistant *Plasmodium falciparum* is an increasing problem in most parts of the world. This has forced the use of combination antimalarial regimes. There is no prophylactic drug treatment for other protozoal infections (right bottom).

Malaria is caused by four species of protozoa (top left) that undergo part of their life cycle in female *Anopheles* mosquitoes. When a mosquito bites a human, it injects sporozoites into a capillary (top left of figure, ●), and these are carried in the blood to the liver, where they multiply and form tissue schizonts. This is the pre-erythrocytic or primary tissue stage of the disease (left half of the figure). After 15–16 days, the schizonts rupture and release (⇨) thousands of merozoites

(●), which infect red blood cells (●) and start the erythrocytic stage of the disease (right figure). In the case of *P. vivax* and *P. ovale* (but not *P. falciparum*), some of the schizonts in the liver remain dormant (▨) and these may rupture months or years later, causing a relapse of the disease (⇨).

Most antimalarials are toxic to the erythrocytic schizonts (blood schizonticides, top right), and the rapidly acting ones (**chloroquine**, **quinine**, **Malarone** [atovaquone with proguanil] and **Riamet** [artemether with lumefantrine]) are used to treat clinical attacks of malaria. **Proguanil** acts too slowly for this purpose and is used to provide prophylaxis. Mefloquine, Malarone and chloroquine are used for both prophylaxis and treatment. However, most *P. falciparum* is now resistant to chloroquine. Quinine is too toxic for prophylaxis. **Primaquine** (left) is a tissue schizonticide used to eliminate the schizonts in the liver (radical cure) once the clinical attack has been controlled.

Blood schizonticides (slow-acting)

Proguanil and **pyrimethamine** are effective schizonticides, but their action is too slow to treat acute attacks. Proguanil is used, usually with chloroquine, for the prophylaxis of malaria. **Proguanil** with **atovaquone** (Malarone) is used to treat resistant *P. falciparum* infections and is increasingly being used by travellers for chemoprophylaxis. Pyrimethamine is given in combination with sulfadoxine (Fansidar) following the use of quinine to treat *P. falciparum* infection. **Sulfadoxine** and **dapsone** act on the same pathway as pyrimethamine, but at a different point (Chapter 37).

Mechanism of action. Pyrimethamine and the active metabolite of proguanil (cycloguanil) are folate antagonists. They inhibit dihydrofolate reductase and, by preventing the regeneration of tetrahydrofolate, they inhibit DNA synthesis and cell division. The drugs are selectively toxic because they have 1000 times the affinity for the plasmodial enzyme than for the human enzyme (compare with methotrexate, Chapter 44, which has a high affinity for the human enzyme).

Blood schizonticides (rapid-acting)

Chloroquine is used to treat *P. vivax* and *P. ovale* infections, but it has no action on the liver schizonts and must be followed by a course of primaquine. In most areas of the world, *P. falciparum* has become resistant to chloroquine, which should not be used for treatment. Chloroquine is usually given orally, but may be given by intravenous infusion to seriously ill patients.

Mechanism of action. Plasmodia within parasitized erythrocytes digest haemoglobin, producing haem (ferriprotoporphyrin IX) that is toxic. Plasmodial haem polymerase converts haem to harmless haemazoin. Chloroquine (and quinine) is concentrated in sensitive plasmodia and inhibits haem polymerase. The resulting accumulation of haem is thought to kill the parasites by a membranolytic action.

Adverse effects. These are unusual with the low doses used for prophylaxis. The higher doses used for treatment may cause nausea, vomiting, diarrhoea, rashes, pruritus and, rarely, psychoses. Prolonged administration of high doses may irreversibly damage the retina.

Quinine, **Malarone** and **Riamet** are used orally to treat *P. falciparum* infections (malignant tertian malaria). Quinine can be given by intravenous infusion if necessary (e.g. unconsciousness). A 7-day course of quinine is given together with, or followed by, **doxycycline** or **clindamycin** or **Fansidar** (pyrimethamine with sulfadoxine). Combined therapy is not necessary with Riamet or Malarone, which are more potent and less toxic than quinine. The mechanism of action of quinine is unknown. Mefloquine is rarely used for treatment of *P. falciparum* because of increased drug resistance.

Adverse effects. Adverse effects of quinine include abdominal pain, nausea, tinnitus, headache, blindness and hypersensitivity reactions. **Mefloquine** may cause neuropsychiatric reactions, and **Malarone** or **doxycycline** is increasingly being used to provide prophylaxis in areas of chloroquine-resistant *P. falciparum*. The main component of Malarone is **atovaquone**, a hydroxynaphthoquinone that acts by inhibiting mitochondrial electron transport in the parasite. **Artemisinin** and its derivatives, e.g. **artemether**, are the most potent and rapidly acting antimalarials. In combination with **lumefantrine**, they are effective against quinine-resistant *P. falciparum*. **Artesunate** with mefloquine is widely used in areas of the world with multidrug-resistant *P. falciparum*, e.g. Thailand.

Tissue schizonticide

Primaquine is an important drug because it is the only antimalarial that will kill the schizonts of *P. vivax* and *P. ovale* lying dormant in the liver. However, it is of no value in treating clinical attacks because it has little effect on the erythrocytic schizonts. The mechanism of action of primaquine is unknown. It seems that oxidative damage to the parasite is caused by active metabolites that may also cause haemolysis of erythrocytes in persons with an inherited deficiency of glucose-6-phosphate dehydrogenase (G6PD). For this reason, the blood of patients should be tested for G6PD activity before starting treatment with primaquine.

Adverse effects include nausea, vomiting, bone marrow depression and haemolytic anaemia.

Other protozoal diseases

Amoebiasis is caused by infection with *Entamoeba histolytica*, a potent pathogen that is the second leading cause of death from parasitic disease. **Metronidazole** (and **tinidazole**) (Chapter 37) are highly effective for treating amoebic colitis and liver abscess. Following a nitroimidazole, all patients are given a luminal agent (**diloxanide** or **paromomycin**) to eliminate cysts.

Giardiasis. *Giardia lamblia* is a flagellate pear-shaped protozoan. It is a common bowel pathogen causing flatulence and diarrhoea. **Metronidazole** is an effective treatment.

Trichomoniasis. *Trichomonas vaginalis* is a common cause of vaginal discharge and occasionally causes urethritis in either gender. **Metronidazole** is usually very effective.

Pneumocystosis. *Pneumocystis carinii* is a common organism that is probably inhaled in early life and lies dormant in the lungs. In immunosuppressed patients (steroids, immunosuppressive drugs, AIDS), it may cause an interstitial pneumonitis. *P. carinii* pneumonia is the most common presentation of AIDS in Western countries. It is treated with **co-trimoxazole** (Chapter 37), **atovaquone** or **pentamidine**. The mechanism of action of pentamidine is unknown, and it has many side-effects, which are sometimes fatal.

Leishmaniasis. The *Leishmania* protozoa are intracellular parasites that are transmitted to humans by the bite of infected sandflies. In most areas, pentavalent antimony (e.g. **stibogluconate**) is the main therapeutic agent for both cutaneous and visceral leishmaniasis. The organic pentavalent antimony compounds react with thiol groups and reduce adenosine triphosphate (ATP) production in the parasite. In most of India, the cure rate with antimony has fallen to 35% and many patients now receive highly effective treatment with **amphotericin** (Chapter 40). **Miltefosine** is the first effective oral treatment for visceral leishmaniasis.

Trypanosomiasis. African trypanosomiasis (sleeping sickness) is spread by the tsetse fly and is caused by infection with either *Trypanosoma gambiense* or *T. rhodesiense*. **Suramin** and **pentamidine** are used before CNS involvement. **Melarsoprol** is used against late-stage disease, but is very toxic. American trypanosomiasis (Chagas disease) is caused by *T. cruzi* carried by triatomine bugs. **Difurtimox** and **benznidazole** are used but do not have high efficacy against chronic disease.

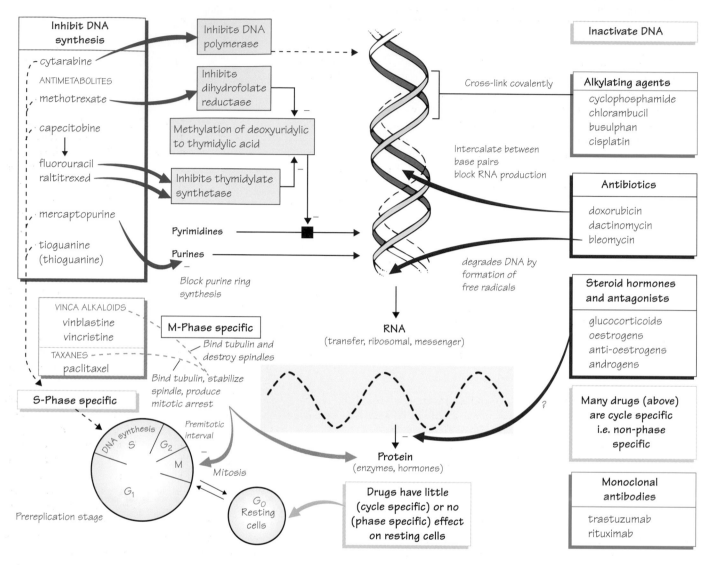

The aim of treatment in patients with cancer is cure or, if this is not possible, effective palliation. Many cancers present as localized tumour masses, but surgery or radiotherapy often fails to eradicate the disease, which eventually becomes widespread. For this reason, there is a trend to incorporate systemic treatment with local treatment at the time of diagnosis.

Drugs used to treat cancer inhibit the mechanisms of cell proliferation. They are therefore toxic to both tumour cells and proliferating normal cells, especially in the *bone marrow*, *gastrointestinal epithelium* and *hair follicles*. The **selectivity** of cytotoxic drugs occurs because, in malignant tumours, a higher proportion of the component cells is undergoing division than in normal proliferating tissues.

Anticancer drugs are classified according to their sites of action along the synthetic pathway of cellular macromolecules (top). Some drugs are only effective during part of the cell cycle (**phase-specific drugs**, left), while others (**cycle-specific drugs**, right) are cytotoxic throughout the cell cycle (lower figure).

Alkylating agents (top right) readily form covalent bonds. They react with the bases in DNA and prevent cell division by cross-linking

the two strands of the double helix. Several **antibiotics** (middle right) isolated from various species of *Streptomyces* also interact with DNA and are widely used as anticancer drugs. Some cytotoxic drugs act by interfering with DNA synthesis (top left). These agents are **antimetabolites** and inhibit purine or pyrimidine synthesis. One is a folic acid antagonist (**methotrexate**). The **vinca alkaloids** and **taxanes** (bottom left) inhibit mitosis by binding to the microtubular proteins necessary for spindle formation. **Monoclonal antibodies** (bottom right) are newer drugs that react with antigen specifically expressed on cancer cells. The Fc portion of the antibody is left exposed and this activates the host's immune mechanism that kills the cancer cells. **Steroid hormones** and hormone antagonists (lower right) are often used in the treatment of cancer. **Combinations** of cytotoxic drugs may be strikingly more successful than single drugs in the treatment of some cancers (e.g. Hodgkin's disease).

The administration of cytotoxic drugs may be associated with unpleasant and even life-threatening **adverse effects**. Individual drugs sometimes have specific toxic effects, but general adverse effects common to many agents include nausea and vomiting (reduced by antiemetics such as metoclopramide, dexamethasone and granisetron), oral and intestinal ulceration, diarrhoea, alopecia and bone marrow suppression, which can decrease the production of any or all of the formed elements of blood. Leucopenia is associated with an increased risk of opportunistic infections; thrombocytopenia leads to bleeding, and decreased red cell formation causes anaemia. **Vincristine** and **bleomycin** are exceptions that do not cause myelosuppression. Most cytotoxic drugs are teratogenic.

Selectivity

The selectivity of antitumour drugs is marginal at best. Their beneficial effects depend on the bone marrow cells recovering faster than the tumour cells after drug administration. Following marrow recovery, more drug can be given and, because a fixed proportion of tumour cells is killed during each period of drug administration, the tumour may eventually be eradicated. **Lenograstim** (recombinant granulocyte colony-stimulating factor) may reduce the duration of drug-induced neutropenia. In practice, the response of tumours to chemotherapy ranges from 'cure', e.g. acute lymphoblastic leukaemia in children, to complete refractoriness, e.g. malignant melanoma.

Alkylating agents

These drugs are widely used in cancer chemotherapy. Prolonged usage often affects gametogenesis severely; most males become permanently sterile. The drugs are associated with an increased incidence of acute non-lymphocytic leukaemia. **Cyclophosphamide** is metabolized in the liver, forming several active metabolites. One metabolite, acrolein, occasionally causes haemorrhagic cystitis, a serious complication. Intravenous administration of 2-*m*ercapto*e*thane *s*ulphonate sodium (*Na*) (mesna) protects the bladder by combining with acrolein in the kidney.

Cytotoxic antibiotics

Doxorubicin is widely used in acute leukaemias, lymphomas and a variety of solid tumours. It is an anthracycline that can slip between neighbouring base pairs in DNA (intercalation). It inhibits DNA and RNA synthesis, probably by an action on topoisomerase II. High cumulative doses are cardiotoxic, probably because oxygen free radicals are formed; these are not inactivated in the heart because it lacks catalase.

Vinca alkaloids and taxanes

Vincristine is used in acute lymphoblastic leukaemia, lymphomas and some solid tumours. It has toxic effects on peripheral and autonomic nerves. **Vinblastine** is used in the treatment of lymphomas and testicular teratomas. It causes more myelosuppression than vincristine, but is less neurotoxic. The taxanes are relatively new drugs derived from bark of yew trees. **Paclitaxel** with cisplatin or carboplatin is the treatment of choice in ovarian cancer. Pretreatment with dexamethasone and antihistamines is necessary to prevent sensitivity reactions.

Antimetabolites

Folic acid antagonists. Methotrexate competitively inhibits dihydrofolate reductase and prevents the regeneration of tetrahydrofolic acid and the coenzyme, methylene tetrahydrofolate, which is essential for the conversion of deoxyuridylic acid to thymidylic acid. Because rapidly dividing cells require an abundant supply of deoxythymidylate for the synthesis of DNA, methotrexate prevents the division of cells. It is used in acute lymphatic leukaemia, lymphomas and several solid tumours.

Antipyrimidines. Fluorouracil is converted to fluorodeoxyuridylic acid, which inhibits thymidylate synthetase, the enzyme responsible for converting deoxyuridylate to thymidylic acid. This impairs DNA synthesis by reducing the availability of thymidylic acid. It is used in the treatment of solid tumours.

Monoclonal antibodies

Trastuzumab targets human epidermal growth factor receptor 2 (HER2/neu) and is used for the treatment of early breast cancer and metastatic breast cancer in patients who over HER2. **Rituximab** lyses B-cell lymphocytes by attaching to a surface protein (CD20). It is used for the treatment of B-cell lymphomas. These drugs are given by intravenous injection and are very toxic. **Bevacizumab** is an inhibitor of vascular endothelial growth factor. It improves survival of patients with colorectal cancer when given with standard treatment, e.g. 5-fluorouracil and folinic acid.

Hormones and hormone antagonists

Glucocorticoids (e.g. **prednisolone**) inhibit cell division by interfering with DNA synthesis. They are widely used in the treatment of leukaemias, lymphomas and breast cancer.

The growth of some tumours, especially carcinoma of the breast and prostate, is partly dependent upon hormones. Removal of the gland producing the hormone (e.g. orchidectomy in prostatic cancer), the administration of hormones with the opposite action, or the administration of an antagonist may induce tumour regression. In women who are steroid hormone receptor-positive, **tamoxifen**, an oestrogen antagonist, is widely used for adjuvant therapy following breast cancer surgery and for the treatment of postmenopausal metastatic breast cancer. Aromatase inhibitors, e.g. **anastrozole** and **letrozole**, block the conversion of androgen to oestrogen in peripheral tissues but not in the ovaries. They should not be used in premenopausal women but are less toxic than, and probably superior to, tamoxifen for the treatment of metastatic breast cancer in postmenopausal women.

In prostatic cancer, **diethylstilbestrol** has been replaced by gonadorelin (synthetic gonadotrophin-releasing hormone [GnRH]) analogues (e.g. **buserelin**), which have fewer adverse effects. When given continuously, GnRH analogues initially stimulate but then inhibit luteinizing hormone (LH) secretion, thereby suppressing testosterone release. The initial increase in LH may cause the tumour to grow. This 'flare' can be prevented with antiandrogens, e.g. **flutamide**. Unfortunately, the effects of hormones are usually temporary, because hormone-independent cells eventually predominate.

Immunosuppressants are used to prevent tissue rejection after organ transplantation, and to treat autoimmune and collagen diseases. **Prednisolone** is widely used, often in combination with **azathioprine** or, in acute rejection, with **mycophenolate mofetil**. **Ciclosporin** and **tacrolimus** are calcineurin inhibitors and potent immunosuppressants that are used with prednisolone. Immunosuppressants have serious adverse effects and, *like cytotoxic drugs*, increase vulnerability to the rapid spread of infections. **Basiliximab** prevents T-lymphocyte proliferation and is used with corticosteroids and ciclosporin to prevent acute rejection of renal transplants.

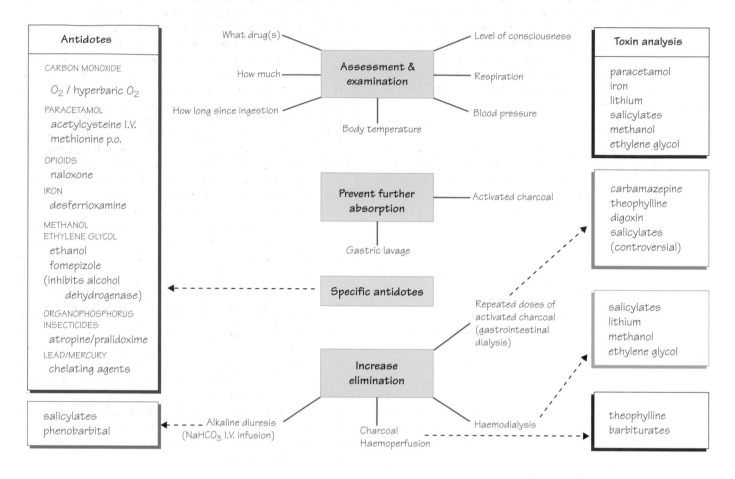

The most common drugs causing death by self-poisoning are **Co-proxamol,*** **paracetamol** alone and **tricyclic antidepressants**. However, the most common cause of fatal self-poisoning, especially in men, is carbon monoxide originating from a car exhaust. Self-poisoning with two or more drugs is not uncommon, and alcohol is also taken in about 50% of incidents. Most cases of intentional self-poisoning are cries for help (parasuicide), but in England and Wales over 3500 people a year successfully kill themselves by poisoning. Once in hospital the mortality of self-poisoners is less than 1%. Accidental self-poisoning occurs mainly in young children (under 5 years) and usually involves medicines or household chemicals (e.g. bleach) left within reach. Patients presenting with poisoning must be given an initial assessment (top) including a rapid but careful clinical examination. It is important to exclude other causes of coma and abnormal behaviour (e.g. head injury, epilepsy, diabetes). Most patients admitted for self-poisoning require only **general supportive measures**. Drug screens are rarely needed as an emergency, but, with some drugs (top right), the clinical state of the patient may not reflect the severity of the overdose, and measurement of the plasma concentration can indicate the use of life-saving techniques (centre bottom) or **specific antidotes** (left).

* Paracetamol + dextropropoxyphene.

Traditionally, routine attempts were made to reduce further absorption of the drug, either by causing emesis with **syrup of ipecacuanha** or by **gastric aspiration** and **lavage**. These time-hallowed treatments are being used less and less because there is no evidence that they improve the outcome in poisoned patients. Increasingly, the oral administration of **activated charcoal** is being used to reduce drug absorption. In volunteer studies, charcoal has been shown to reduce the absorption of many drugs, especially in the first hour after administration. Unfortunately, clinical studies have failed to show that charcoal affects the outcome of poisoning. Nevertheless, charcoal is often given to patients who have ingested a potentially toxic amount of poison within the previous hour. Techniques used to **increase drug elimination** (bottom) have a limited role, but are important in a small number of severely poisoned patients.

Reduction of absorption

Emesis
Syrup of ipecacuanha induces emesis in over 90% of patients. It can only be used in conscious patients. There is no evidence that ipecacuanha reduces the severity of poisoning and its use has been abandoned.

Gastric aspiration and lavage

An orogastric tube is passed into the stomach, which is then washed out with 300–600 mL of water (three or four times or until the effluent is clear). If the patient is unconscious, the airway must be protected with a cuffed endotracheal tube. After an hour from ingestion, lavage removes only a tiny proportion of the poison and there is no evidence that the procedure is beneficial. Early lavage (within 60 min of ingestion) may benefit patients who have taken a potentially life-threatening amount of poison. Gastric lavage is contraindicated in poisoning with corrosives or petroleum compounds.

Activated charcoal

Activated charcoal is a very fine porous black powder with an enormous surface area in relation to mass ($1000 \ m^2 \ g^{-1}$). It binds many drugs, and 10 g of charcoal will absorb about 1 g of drug. Charcoal does not absorb iron, lithium, corrosive agents or organic solvents. Charcoal is contraindicated in patients with an unprotected airway (e.g. drowsy or comatose patients) because there is a risk of pulmonary aspiration.

Enhancement of elimination

Enhancement of elimination can reduce the time of recovery, but there is little evidence that it changes morbidity, except in severely comatose patients (grade IV coma).

Repeated doses of activated charcoal. Repeated oral doses of charcoal may increase elimination by gastrointestinal dialysis; it has the merit of being relatively safe (unless aspirated).

Alkaline diuresis. The urine is made alkaline (pH 7.5–8.5) by the administration of $NaHCO_3$ (intravenous infusion). This ionizes weak acids, e.g. aspirin, in the renal tubules and reduces reabsorption. Similarly, acid diuresis may be useful in cases of poisoning with basic drugs such as amfetamine and 'ecstasy'. Forced alkaline diuresis using large intravenous volumes of water containing $NaHCO_3$ is hazardous and is no longer used.

Haemodialysis and haemoperfusion are invasive techniques requiring cannulation of an artery and vein (usually in the arm) to establish a temporary extracorporeal circulation. In haemodialysis, the drug passes down its concentration gradient through the dialysis membrane and is removed in the dialysis fluid. In haemoperfusion, the blood is passed through a column of activated charcoal or resin onto which the drug is absorbed. These techniques have significant risks (haemorrhage, air embolism, infection, loss of a peripheral artery) and the shortened elimination half-life does not necessarily correlate with improved clinical state (i.e. reduced morbidity or mortality). In some cases, e.g. carbamazepine poisoning, multiple doses of activated charcoal are as effective as haemoperfusion.

Aspirin

The symptoms of salicylate poisoning include tinnitus, hyperventilation and sweating. Coma is uncommon and indicates very severe poisoning. Acid–base disturbances are complicated because aspirin stimulates the respiratory centre, causing a respiratory alkalosis, but also uncouples oxidative phosphorylation, which may cause a metabolic acidosis. Immediate management includes measurement of plasma salicylate concentration (at 4–6 h post-ingestion), electrolytes and blood gases. Gastric lavage (up to 1 h after ingestion) is followed by activated charcoal administration. Severe poisoning (plasma concentration above 500 mg L^{-1}) requires urinary alkalinization. In very severe poisoning, haemodialysis is the treatment of choice.

Paracetamol

Initially, patients may be asymptomatic or complain only of nausea and vomiting. But, after a delay of 48–72 h, relatively small amounts (more than 10 g, 20–30 tablets) may cause fatal hepatocellular necrosis. Normally, paracetamol is metabolized, mainly by conjugation reactions in the liver, but high doses saturate these pathways and the drug is then oxidized to a reactive (toxic) quinone intermediate (*N*-acetylbenzoquinoneimine). The quinone can be inactivated by combination with glutathione, but high doses of paracetamol deplete the hepatic glutathione stores and the reactive quinone then covalently binds to thiol groups on the cell proteins and kills the cell. **Acetylcysteine** (intravenous or oral) and **methionine** (oral) are potentially life-saving antidotes in cases of paracetamol poisoning because they increase the synthesis of liver glutathione. Patients who have taken an overdose of paracetamol should have a blood sample taken at 4 h (or later) after ingestion to determine quickly the plasma concentration of drug so that the antidote can be given. If less than 1 h has elapsed since ingestion, a dose of activated charcoal should be given. The decision on whether to continue treatment with the antidote is decided by referring the plasma paracetamol concentration to a graph that joins plots of 200 mg L^{-1} at 4 h and 6.5 mg L^{-1} at 24 h. This graph is based on outcome studies of many fatal and non-fatal cases of poisoning carried out before effective treatment became available. If the patient's drug concentration is above this 'normal treatment line', antidote treatment is continued. Patients taking enzyme-inducing drugs (including alcohol) and those with glutathione depletion (e.g. patients with eating disorders) are at increased risk; for these patients the antidote is given if the plasma concentration of paracetamol is above a lower 'high-risk line'. If the time since ingestion is less than 4 h, the plasma concentration is unreliable because paracetamol absorption will be continuing. The most effective antidote is acetylcysteine given intravenously within 8 h of paracetamol ingestion. Adverse effects, including anaphylactoid reactions, occur in about 5% of patients.

Opioids

Opioids cause coma, pinpoint pupils and respiratory depression. They are specifically antagonized by **naloxone**, which is given intravenously in repeated doses until ventilation is adequate. Naloxone has a shorter half-life than most opioids and toxicity may recur, necessitating further doses. Naloxone may cause an acute withdrawal syndrome in opioid addicts.

Tricyclic antidepressants

Toxicity following overdosage arises mainly from central anticholinergic effects (respiratory depression, hallucinations, convulsions) and cardiotoxicity. Most patients require only observation or simple supportive measures, such as oxygen to correct hypoxia and activated charcoal (within 1 h). The most common arrhythmia is sinus tachycardia as a result of an atropine-like effect. Lengthening of the QRS complex (a quinidine-like effect) is an ominous sign and may presage convulsions, which may be controlled by intravenous **diazepam** or **clomethiazole**. Prolonged QRS or arrhythmias are treated with intravenous sodium bicarbonate. The use of gastric lavage in tricyclic poisoning is controversial because the gastric contents may be pushed beyond the pylorus and increase the amount of drug absorbed. Struggle during lavage may cause hypoxia and provoke life-threatening arrhythmias.

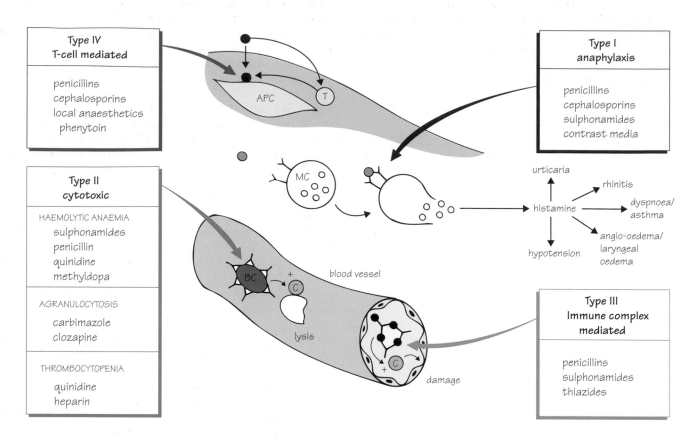

The incidence of adverse (harmful) drug reactions is difficult to establish, but up to 5% of acute admissions to hospital result from an adverse reaction to drugs given in general practice. In hospital, up to 20% of patients experience an adverse drug reaction, and although these are rarely life-threatening, they account for 0.5–1% of hospital inpatient deaths. It has been estimated that, in the USA, adverse drug reactions cause over 100 000 deaths each year, making them the fourth most common cause of death.

The majority of adverse drug reactions can be divided into those that are **dose related** and those that are **non-dose related**; the latter, which occur less frequently, often have an immunological basis. A few drugs are associated with an increased incidence of birth defects (**teratogens**) or tumours (**carcinogens**). Some drugs, when given continuously, lead to **adaptive changes**, and stopping the drug causes unwanted withdrawal effects (e.g. benzodiazepines – insomnia and anxiety; corticosteroids – acute adrenal insufficiency).

Dose-related (type A) adverse drug reactions are predictable and are caused by an excess of the drug's desired pharmacological effect (e.g. hypoglycaemia with insulin, bleeding with heparin) or sometimes a drug's parallel unwanted action (e.g. respiratory depression with morphine). Dose-related adverse drug reactions occur most often with drugs that have a steep dose–response curve and/or a small difference between therapeutic and toxic doses (i.e. a low **therapeutic index = toxic dose/therapeutic dose**). Commonly used drugs with a **low therapeutic index** include *anticoagulants, hypoglycaemic drugs, digoxin,*

antiarrhythmics, aminoglycosides, xanthines, cytotoxic and *immunosuppressive drugs.* Dose-related adverse drug reactions are usually caused by *incorrect dosage* (too high) or *altered pharmacokinetics,* usually impaired drug elimination (e.g. renal failure). **Drug interactions** are involved in 10–20% of adverse drug reactions and are especially common in the elderly, who are more likely to receive multiple drugs for multiple ailments.

Non-dose-related (idiosyncratic, type B) adverse drug reactions are relatively rare, but are unpredictable and, in contrast to dose-related adverse drug reactions, have a considerable mortality. Drug allergy may involve hypersensitivity reactions (types I–IV, figure), but others are not easily classified. Anaphylaxis is the most common serious drug allergy and is potentially fatal.

Dose-related (type A) adverse reactions

Pharmacokinetic variations

The elimination of drugs is very variable in normal individuals, and genetic factors can reduce drug elimination and cause adverse reactions (e.g. succinylcholine causes prolonged apnoea in patients with defective pseudocholinesterase, Chapter 4). **Renal disease** can lead to accumulation and toxicity if a drug is excreted by glomerular filtration or tubular secretion (e.g. gentamicin and other aminoglycosides, digoxin, amphotericin, captopril).

Drug interactions

Drug interaction is the modification of the action of one drug by another and involves **pharmacodynamic** or **pharmacokinetic** mechanisms. Drugs with steep dose–response curves and serious dose-related toxicities are especially likely to be involved in adverse drug interactions (i.e. those with a low therapeutic index, opposite page).

Pharmacodynamic interactions

Pharmacodynamic interactions are the most common and usually have a simple mechanism. Thus, drugs with similar actions, e.g. benzodiazepines and alcohol, produce additive effects and may cause severe central nervous system depression. Conversely, drugs may have opposite actions; e.g. in asthmatic patients β-blockers will oppose β-agonists (and theophylline) and may precipitate severe or even fatal asthma.

Pharmacokinetic interactions

Absorption Drugs that increase (e.g. metoclopramide) or decrease (e.g. atropine) the rate of gastric emptying may affect absorption. Enterohepatic recirculation of oral contraceptives (especially low-dose oestrogen) may be decreased by antibiotics and lead to pregnancy (antibiotics kill the gut bacteria that normally release the steroid from the conjugated form excreted in bile).

Distribution Many drugs are bound to plasma albumin and may be displaced by a second drug. With the exception of a few drugs (e.g. warfarin, phenytoin, tolbutamide), which are more than 90% bound, the displacement of drugs by this mechanism is usually of little practical consequence because increased elimination quickly reduces the plasma concentration of free drug to its original value.

Metabolism Induction of hepatic enzymes by a second drug (e.g. phenytoin, phenobarbital, carbamazepine, rifampicin) can decrease the efficacy of drugs metabolized by the same enzymes (e.g. warfarin). Enzyme inhibitors (e.g. cimetidine) potentiate the effects of warfarin and may cause phenytoin and theophylline toxicity. Other examples are discussed in Chapter 4.

Excretion Drugs may share the same transport system in the proximal tubules. Thus, probenecid competitively reduces penicillin excretion. Thiazide and loop diuretics reduce sodium reabsorption, causing a compensatory increase in the reabsorption of monovalent ions in the proximal tubule. This process can result in lithium accumulation and severe toxicity in patients receiving lithium therapy. Potassium-sparing diuretics combined with potassium supplements and/or angiotensin converting enzyme (ACE) inhibitors cause hyperkalaemia.

Non-dose-related (idiosyncratic, type B) adverse reactions

Hypersensitivity reactions to drugs (drug allergy) involve immunological reactions. Large molecules, e.g. vaccines, insulin and dextrans, can themselves be immunogenic, but most drugs are small molecules and are not antigenic on their own. In some patients (we do not know which), a drug, or a metabolite, acts as a hapten and combines with tissue proteins, forming an antigenic conjugate. The antigens induce the synthesis of antibodies and subsequent exposure to the drug triggers an immunological reaction (e.g. rash, anaphylaxis). Although drug allergy is unpredictable, it is more likely to occur in patients with a history of atopic disease (hay fever, asthma, eczema).

Anaphylaxis is a **type I reaction** in which the drug (●) interacts with IgE fixed to mast cells (MC) and basophils, triggering the release of histamine and other mediators (Chapter 11). Drugs likely to cause this life-threatening reaction (top right) include penicillin, which is responsible for 75% of all anaphylactic deaths. Some drugs (e.g. some contrast media) can produce an anaphylaxis-like (anaphylactoid) reaction on first exposure.

Blood dyscrasias. Allergic reactions to drugs that cause blood dyscrasias (bottom left) involve **type II cytotoxic reactions**. Circulating antibody of the IgM or IgG type interacts with a drug (hapten) combined with the blood cell membrane to form an antigenic complex (—◅). Complement (ⓒ) is activated, causing cell lysis. Some drugs predictably cause blood dyscrasias. For example, most cytotoxic anticancer agents (Chapter 44) inhibit cell division in the bone marrow, and patients with glucose-6-phosphate dehydrogenase deficiency have a high risk of haemolytic anaemia if given primaquine (Chapter 43).

Serum sickness is a **type III reaction** triggered by some drugs (bottom right), where antibody (IgG) combines with the hapten–protein–antigen complex in the circulation. The resulting complex, instead of being removed normally by phagocytic cells, remains in the tissues or circulation. Phagocytic cells and complement (ⓒ) are activated, causing inflammation and damage to the capillary endothelium. This is especially serious when the complexes are stuck to walls of vital blood vessels (e.g. renal glomeruli). The symptoms include fever, arthritis, urticaria and lymphadenopathy.

Rashes. Drugs (top left) cause a wide variety of rashes, some of which are life-threatening but fortunately rare, e.g. toxic epidermal necrolysis (35% mortality). **Type IV cell-mediated reactions** are involved in which T-lymphocytes (Ⓣ) are sensitized by a hapten–protein complex. When the lymphocytes come into contact with the antigen-presenting cell (APC), an inflammatory response is produced. If the antigen (●) enters through the skin (e.g. antibiotic cream), contact sensitivity may cause an eczematous rash with oedema at the application site.

Teratogenesis

Teratogenesis is the occurrence of fetal developmental abnormalities caused by drugs taken during the first trimester of pregnancy. Most drugs cross the placental barrier to some extent and, if possible, drugs should be avoided during pregnancy. Known teratogens include alcohol (fetal alcohol syndrome), anticancer drugs, warfarin (multiple congenital defects), valproate, carbamazepine (neural tube defects) and other anticonvulsants and tetracyclines (inhibition of bone growth).

Carcinogenesis

Drug-induced tumours are probably very rare because the pharmaceutical industry makes great efforts to avoid marketing carcinogenic agents. The mechanisms involved in chemical carcinogenesis are usually unknown, but immunosuppression (e.g. azathioprine with prednisolone) is associated with a greatly increased risk of lymphomas. Alkylating agents (e.g. cyclophosphamide) are thought to exhibit 'gene toxicity' and may cause non-lymphocytic leukaemias.

Case studies and questions

Case 1 Deliberate poisoning

A poisonous gas is released in the London underground. Passengers are brought to the surface by emergency workers in protective clothing. The surviving passengers are sweating, have pinpoint pupils, bradycardia, difficulty in breathing, and are salivating copiously. Some start to have convulsions.

1 *What type of agent was released?*
2 *What is the mechanism of the poisoning?*
3 *What should be done?*

Case 2 Adverse drug effect

A 40-year-old man is given an intravenous injection of penicillin for pneumonia. A few minutes later, he is found with profound hypotension, is dyspnoeic with wheezing and has an urticarial rash.

1 *What has happened to this patient?*
2 *What mechanisms are involved?*
3 *Outline the appropriate treatment of this patient.*

Case 3 Duodenal ulcer

A 62-year-old man complains of epigastric pain that is worse with fasting and better after food. He has found that the pain is relieved by antacids. A tentative diagnosis of duodenal ulcer is confirmed by endoscopy. A ^{13}C-urea breath test (Chapter 12) indicates *Helicobacter pylori* infection.

1 *Should the patient be given treatment to eradicate* H. pylori?
2 *If so, what drugs would you prescribe?*
3 *What treatment might you give to heal the ulcer?*
4 *A year later, the patient develops arthritis and requires NSAIDs to control the pain. How could you minimize the risk of the NSAID treatment inducing further ulcers?*

Case 4 Hypertension

A routine blood pressure measurement at a GP surgery revealed that the patient, a 50-year-old man, had a blood pressure of 180/110. Several repeated visits confirmed these pressures. No cause was found for the hypertension although the patient smoked 20 cigarettes a day and was slightly obese.

1 *At this time, the patient felt perfectly well and asked why he should be worried about his blood pressure. What will you tell him?*
2 *What general advice will you give?*
3 *What antihypertensive drug might you consider for initial therapy?*
4 *After 3 months his blood pressure is still not controlled. What factors might be contributing to this failure of treatment and what should you do next?*

Case 5 Myocardial infarction

A 60-year-old man is brought to A&E with central crushing chest pain. He has been in pain for several hours and it was not relieved by nitroglycerin. The man was feeling nauseous and was very anxious. His blood pressure was 140/75. An ECG revealed ST segment elevation, pathological Q waves and inversion of the T wave in leads II, III and aVF. A diagnosis of acute inferior myocardial infarction (MI) was made.

1 *What drugs should be administered immediately to this patient?*
2 *What contraindications should you consider?*

3 *What drugs would you prescribe for this patient to take long-term when he returns home?*

Case 6 Atrial fibrillation and congestive heart failure

A man aged 72 years is found to have atrial fibrillation. He is prescribed digoxin to control the ventricular response rate. Blood test results at the time included: Na$^+$ 135 mmol/L (133–148), K$^+$ 4.0 mmol/L (3.4–5.3), creatinine 145 μmol/L (45–120), urea 15 mmol/L (2.5–7.0). Three years later, he has gained weight and has swollen ankles. He is also short of breath on minimal exertion and is waking up at night severely breathless. Congestive heart failure is diagnosed and the patient is prescribed bendroflumethazide and enalapril. His symptoms improve but within a year he is brought to hospital where he is found to be in complete heart block. Blood tests reveal: Na$^+$ 140 mmol/L, K$^+$ 2.2 mmol/L, creatinine 370 μmol/L, urea 45 mmol/L.

1 *How does digoxin control the ventricular rate?*
2 *What did the first blood tests indicate?*
3 *What did the second blood tests indicate? What might have caused the changes in blood chemistry?*
4 *Can any of the changes in blood chemistry be responsible for the heart block and if so describe the mechanisms involved.*

Case 7 Insomnia

An 85-year-old man is given diazepam to help him sleep at night. A few weeks later his son finds him in a state of self-neglect. He is taken to hospital where he is found to be drowsy and confused.

1 *Why was diazepam a bad choice of drug for this elderly patient?*
2 *How should he be treated in hospital?*
3 *What would be a more suitable hypnotic for this patient?*

Case 8 Drug abuse

A 20-year-old man is found unconscious in a park. He is brought to A&E. There are no signs of injury and his blood sugar is normal. A used syringe was found by him and there are needle tracks on his arms. He has small pupils and slow, shallow respiration.

1 *What is the most likely diagnosis?*
2 *What treatment should be given immediately?*
3 *The patient recovers consciousness but an hour later becomes unconscious again. What has happened?*

Case 9 Suicide attempt

A young man arrives at A&E. He has recently broken up with his girlfriend and decided to kill himself. He swallowed a number of paracetamol (acetaminophen) tablets but 3 or 4 hours later decided that he did not, after all, want to commit suicide. When questioned about the number of tablets taken, he is rather uncertain, but thinks he has taken about 30.

Apart from feeling nauseous, the man lacks other significant symptoms.

1 *Should this patient be given activated charcoal?*
2 *Five hours after ingestion, the plasma concentration of paracetamol is found to be 230 mg/L. How does this value help in assessing the risk of liver damage in this patient?*
3 *You decide the patient is at risk of liver damage. What antidote would you administer? What test could you use to monitor liver damage caused by paracetamol?*

4 *What is the mechanism of paracetamol hepatotoxicity and how does the antidote work?*

5 *Which patients suffering from paracetamol poisoning are at particularly high risk of liver damage? How would you treat these high-risk patients?*

Case 10 Collapse

A 60-year-old man with stable angina pectoris has been having an affair with a younger woman for several months. Worried about his sexual performance, he purchased sildenafil (Viagra) from an internet pharmacy. At his most recent visit to his mistress he took a Viagra tablet but whilst waiting for the expected beneficial effects he lost consciousness and collapsed onto the floor.

1 *How does sildenafil produce its beneficial effects in men with erectile dysfunction?*

2 *What is the most likely cause of the man's collapse?*

3 *How would you treat this man and what advice would you give him for the future?*

Answers

Case 1 Deliberate poisoning

1 An organophosphorus anticholinesterase, e.g. sarin.

2 These agents are absorbed through the bronchi and skin, therefore contaminated clothing should be removed and the skin washed. Organophosphorus anticholinesterases inhibit cholinesterases irreversibly and cause acetylcholine (ACh) to accumulate in cholinergic synapses. The resulting stimulation of the parasympathetic nervous system causes most of the symptoms of the victims. Nicotinic effects may also occur, e.g. muscle fasciculation, flaccid paralysis (due to depolarizing neuromuscular block, cf. succinylcholine, Chapter 6). Organophosphorus anticholinesterases readily pass the blood–brain barrier and may cause central effects, e.g. convulsions.

3 **Atropine** is given by intravenous or intramuscular injection every 5–10 min to control the muscarinic effects. The dose depends on the severity of the poisoning and is increased until the pupils dilate, the skin becomes flushed, and tachycardia develops.

Pralidoxime. Organophosphorus anticholinesterases inactivate the enzyme by phosphorylating the serine hydroxyl group. Little or no hydrolysis of the phosphorylated enzyme occurs and the agents are essentially irreversible. Pralidoxime reactivates the enzyme because it has an oxime group that preferentially bonds with the organophosphorus anticholinesterase.

Diazepam may be necessary to control convulsions.

Case 2 Adverse drug effect

1 The patient is suffering from anaphylactic shock.

2 Anaphylaxis is a type I allergic reaction (Chapter 46) in which the drug interacts with IgE fixed to mast cells and basophils causing the release of histamine, leukotrienes and other mediators. Histamine causes vasodilatation and hypotension and increases the permeability of capillaries. Leakage of plasma from the capillaries causes swelling of the soft tissues (angio-oedema), and if the larynx is involved the swelling may be life-threatening. Histamine also impairs respiration by causing bronchoconstriction.

3 Treatment must be prompt. Epinephrine (adrenaline) is given by intramuscular or slow intravenous injection to raise the blood pressure and dilate the bronchi. Oxygen is given to reduce hypoxia. Following the epinephrine, an H_1-antihistamine (e.g. chlorphenamine) and hydrocortisone are administered by intramuscular or intravenous injection. The hydrocortisone reduces vascular permeability and suppresses any further response to the antigen–antibody reaction. Hydrocortisone takes several hours to act (Chapter 33). In severe anaphylaxis, the leaky capillaries lead to a reduction of circulating volume and the rapid infusion of plasma substitute is necessary.

Penicillins account for 75% of anaphylactic reactions to drugs. Other agents especially associated with anaphylaxis include other antibacterials, vaccines, blood products, NSAIDs and heparin. Anaphylaxis, especially in atopic individuals, may be caused by insect stings and certain foods, e.g. fish, cow's milk, eggs and peanuts.

Case 3 Duodenal ulcer

1 Yes, successful eradication of *H. pylori* infection usually results in long-term remission of the ulcer.

2 Inhibition of acid secretion with a proton-pump inhibitor (e.g. omeprazole) in combination with two antibacterials (e.g. clarithromycin and metronidazole or amoxicillin) can eradicate *H. pylori* in over 90% of patients in 7 days. Reinfection is rare. (See Chapter 12 for connection between *H. pylori* infection and acid secretion.)

3 Ulcer-healing drugs either reduce acid secretion (proton-pump inhibitors, histamine H_2-receptor antagonists) or protect the gastric mucosa (sucralfate, bismuth, misoprostol). Following the successful eradication of *H. pylori*, it is not usually necessary to use these drugs unless the ulcer is large or complicated by haemorrhage.

4 Gastric or duodenal ulcers occur in 1–5% of patients taking NSAIDs, the incidence increasing greatly in those over 60 years of age. The patient here is 60 years old and has a significant risk of ulceration. This can be minimized by giving an NSAID that is a non-selective COX-inhibitor (e.g. ibuprofen) in combination with either misoprostol or a proton-pump inhibitor. An alternative would be to give a selective COX-2 inhibitor (e.g. celecoxib), but these drugs are associated with an increased incidence of myocardial infarction and stroke (Chapter 32).

Case 4 Hypertension

1 That his high blood pressure increases his risk of coronary artery disease, heart failure, renal failure, and stroke.

2 Stress the importance of giving up smoking. Suggest that he loses weight by eating less and taking more exercise. Also suggest a reduction in alcohol consumption and avoidance of added salt as both of these may be contributory factors involved in his hypertension.

3 The main drugs used to treat hypertension are the thiazides, angiotensin-converting enzyme inhibitors (ACEIs), angiotensin-II receptor antagonists (ARAs) and calcium channel blockers (CCBs). The response to ACEIs and ARAs is often reduced in patients over the age of 55 years probably because they have lower renin levels than younger patients. Therefore, a thiazide (e.g. bendroflumethiazide) or CCB (e.g. amlodipine) would be a reasonable choice.

4 The most likely explanation for the failure to control the patient's blood pressure is lack of compliance. Tactful questions may reveal that the drug selected for initial therapy has unwanted effects that the patient finds unacceptable. If you are convinced the patient is taking his medicine as directed, then a second drug should be added. For patients taking a thiazide or CCB, the addition of an ACEI (e.g. captopril) or ARA (losartan) is appropriate because both diuresis and vasodilatation stimulate the renin-angiotensin system and turn non-renin-dependent hypertension into renin-dependent hypertension. Some patients may require three or even four drugs to control their hypertension. Multidrug therapy is likely to reduce compliance but this can be improved by the use of sustained-release formulations and fixed-dose combinations (e.g. Co-zidocapt, which is captopril in combination with hydrochlorothiazide).

Case 5 Myocardial infarction

1 Aspirin is given to reduce further platelet aggregation. Oxygen is administered, and intravenous diamorphine together with an antiemetic (e.g. metoclopramide) is given to reduce the pain. A nitrate (e.g. glyceryl trinitrate, isosorbide dinitrate) may reduce the work of the heart and help to control the ischaemic pain. A β-blocker (e.g. propranolol) should be given. β-Blockers reduce the rate and the oxygen demand of the heart and decrease ventricular wall stress by lowering the afterload.

When given acutely, β-blockers reduce ischaemia and infarct size. They also suppress arrhythmias (Chapter 17).

Revascularization. A thrombolytic agent (e.g. streptokinase, tissue plasminogen activator [tPA], Chapter 19) should be administered to dissolve the thrombus and restore patency of the occluded artery. Clinical trials have shown that in MI with ST segment elevation, thrombolytic drugs reduce mortality by 25%. It is important that the drug is given as soon as possible, ideally within 1 h, although significant reductions in mortality occur up to 12 h from the onset of symptoms. tPA, reteplase and tenecteplase are more fibrin specific than streptokinase, and intravenous heparin is used for 48–72 h as adjunctive therapy to prevent re-thrombosis. Increasingly, primary percutaneous intervention (PCI), to mechanically disrupt the occlusion within the culprit epicardial coronary artery, is replacing pharmacological thrombolysis (see Chapter 19).

2 The drugs cited above have the following contraindications:
Aspirin: allergy, history of active peptic ulceration.
β-Blocker: left ventricular failure.
Thrombolytics: recent haemorrhage, cerebrovascular disease (e.g. stroke), uncontrolled hypertension, and in the case of streptokinase, previous allergic reaction. Antibodies to streptokinase develop and reduce its effectiveness. For this reason it should not be used beyond 4 days of first administration.

3 The long-term management of this patient involves the use of a number of drugs. Glyceryl trinitrate for anginal pain. To prevent platelet aggregation, aspirin should be given together with Clopidogrel. Warfarin is occasionally used in patients with extensive myocardial infarction or evidence of blood clots in the left ventricle. A β-blocker should be prescribed because long-term use has been shown to reduce mortality, recurrent MI and sudden death by about 25%. Treatment with an ACE-inhibitor should be started within 24 hours and continued when the patient is discharged, especially if there is evidence of left ventricular dysfunction. ACE-inhibitors reduce afterload and improve ejection fraction. They also reduce ventricular remodelling and infarct expansion, actions that reduce mortality, the incidence of heart failure, and further MIs. The patient should be given a statin (Chapter 20) because they have been shown to reduce the incidence of coronary events.

Case 6 Atrial fibrillation and congestive heart failure

1 In addition to its direct effects on the heart, digoxin acts centrally and stimulates vagal activity, increasing ACh release from parasympathetic nerve endings in the heart. This slows atrioventricular conductance and prolongs the refractory period of the atrioventricular node. The atrial arrthythmia is unaffected but the ventricular rate is slowed, allowing improved ventricular filling and pumping efficiency.

2 Renal impairment.

3 The blood tests show a deterioration in renal function. This could be due to an adverse effect of the enalapril. ACE inhibitors may impair renal function by reducing glomerular filling pressure or causing glomerulonephritis. This patient's plasma creatine levels should have been measured after initiation and regularly during his treatment.

4 Digoxin is cleared mainly by the kidneys. In this patient raised creatine and urea plasma levels indicate renal impairment. This may have reduced the clearance of digoxin to such an extent that the plasma concentration of drug reached toxic levels. The patient also has hypokalaemia, probably caused by the diuretic (Chapter 14). Potassium competes for digoxin at the site of action of the drug on the cardiac muscle Na^+/K^+-ATPase. Thus, a low plasma concentration of K^+ increases the action of digoxin, causing adverse effects such as the heart block that occurred in this patient.

Case 7 Insomnia

1 Diazepam is slowly eliminated and has active metabolites that are even more slowly eliminated. Elderly patients may have subclinical hepatic or renal impairment, causing the benzodiazepines to accumulate. This results in 'hangover' effects during the day. These include confusion and ataxia, which may result in falls and injury.

2 The diazepam should be stopped. Flumazenil is a specific antagonist of drugs that act on benzodiazepine receptors and may be used in benzodiazepine overdosage where there is respiratory depression. Flumazenil is not without risk, e.g. in patients dependent on benzodiazepines, and is not indicated in this patient.

3 A short-acting benzodiazepine, e.g. temazepam, or a 'Z-drug', e.g. zolpidem (Chapter 24), may be used for a short period (not more than a few weeks at most). Elderly patients are often more sensitive to central depressants than younger patients and the hypnotic should be given at a reduced dose.

Case 8 Drug abuse

1 Opioid overdose (probably heroin but addicts will inject any opioid available).

2 Naloxone is a specific antagonist at opioid receptors and is the antidote given by intravenous injection in cases of opioid overdose.

3 Naloxone has a shorter duration of action than many opioids. The naloxone has probably been cleared, allowing the effects of the opioid to reappear. Patients given naloxone require careful monitoring as repeated injections may be necessary to prevent respiratory depression. Some opioids (e.g. methadone) have a very long durations of action.

Case 9 Suicide attempt

1 No, it's too late. Activated charcoal is only worthwhile if administered within 1 h of paracetamol ingestion.

2 Providing it is at least 4 h since the ingestion of paracetamol, the plasma concentration of drug can be used to assess the likelihood of liver damage by using a plot of paracetamol concentration against time (see British National Formulary and Chapter 45). The normogram below is based on outcome studies of many fatal and non-fatal cases of poisoning carried out before effective treatment became available. If the plasma concentration is above the normal treatment line, as it is in this patient, then the antidote is administered.

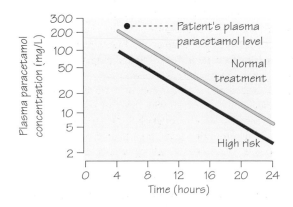

3 *N*-Acetylcysteine (NAC) is an effective antidote, and intravenous infusion given within 24 h protects the liver from damage. NAC is most

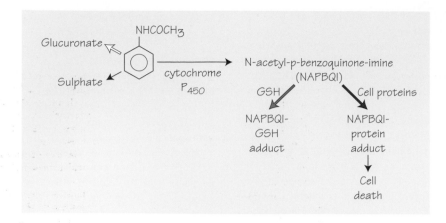

effective if administered within 8 h but treatment continuing for up to 72 h may provide benefit. If NAC is unavailable, oral methionine is also effective but administration is difficult if the patient is vomiting.

The international normalized ratio (INR: ratio of prothrombin time to normal prothrombin time) is a sensitive measure used to monitor liver damage.

4 Paracetamol (acetaminophen) is *N*-acetyl-*p*-aminophenol.

Normal doses of paracetamol are metabolized to glucuronate and sulphate. However, high doses saturate these processes and P450 mixed function oxidases produce a toxic metabolite, *N*-acetyl-*p*-benzoquinone imine (NAPBQI). This may be inactivated by conjugation with gluta-thione (GSH) (←) but toxic doses deplete the GSH stores and NAPBQI then reacts with cell proteins (→). This causes hepatocellular necrosis and, much more rarely, renal tubular necrosis. Regeneration of GSH requires cysteine, the availability of which can be limiting. NAC and methionine can substitute for cysteine and by increasing the synthesis of GSH they divert the reaction of NAPBQI away from cell proteins.

5 Enzyme-inducing drugs (Chapter 14) increase the toxicity of para-cetamol. When patients are taking these drugs, the plasma paracetamol concentration is referred to the high-risk line on the plot of paracetamol concentration against time. This line is below the normal treatment line and indicates administration of NAC or methionine at lower concentra-tions of paracetamol. The high-risk line is also used for malnourished patients, e.g. anorexics and alcoholics.

Case 10 Collapse

1 Penile erection depends on nitric oxide (NO) release from nitrergic nerves and vascular endothelial cells. NO raises the intracellular concentration of cGMP in the smooth muscle of the arteries, arterioles and trabeculae of the erectile tissue. The resulting smooth muscle relaxation increases penile blood flow and quickly leads to filling of the sinusoids and expansion of the corpora cavernosa. This compresses the venous plexuses between the trabeculae and the firm tunica albuginea occluding the venous outflow and causing erection. The action of cGMP is terminated by phosphodiesterase-5 (PDE5), an isoenzyme of PDE that is present in penile vascular smooth muscle. Sildenafil is a selective inhibitor of PDE5, and by prolonging the action of cGMP improves the erectile response to sexual stimulation.

2 The man was probably taking an organic nitrate for prophylaxis of his angina pectoris. Nitrates cause vasodilatation by producing NO and increasing intracellular cGMP levels in vascular smooth muscle (Chapter 16). Sildenafil inhibits the vascular cGMP and potentiates the action of nitrates causing severe, and potentially fatal hypotension. A rapid fall in blood pressure probably resulted in the collapse of this unfortunate man.

3 The man should be placed in a supine position with his legs raised to restore venous return to the heart. He should be informed that Viagra interacts dangerously with the medicine he is taking for his angina. He might usefully be advised to consult his doctor before self-prescribing any further drugs.

Index

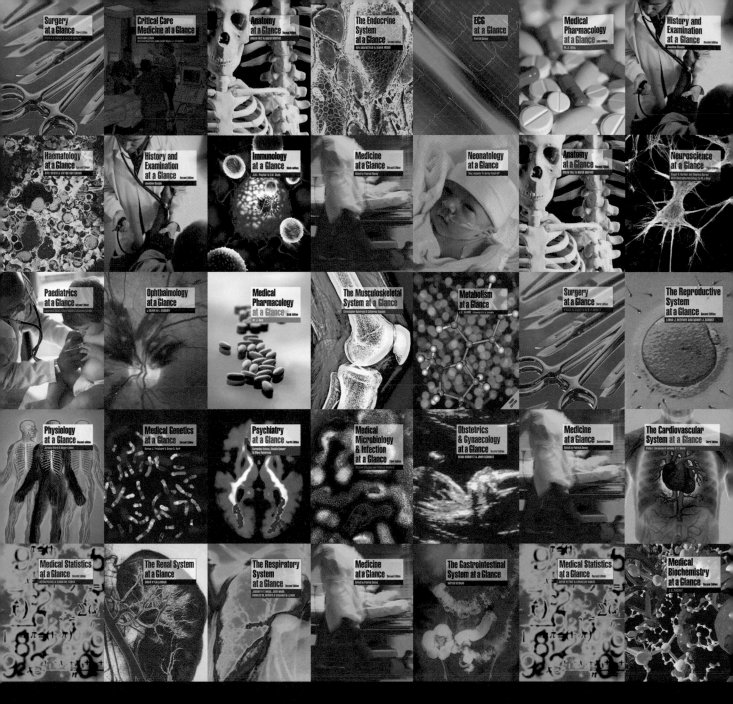

The at a Glance series

Popular double-page spread format · Coverage of core knowledge

Full-colour throughout · Self-assessment to test your knowledge · Expert authors

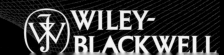

WILEY-
BLACKWELL

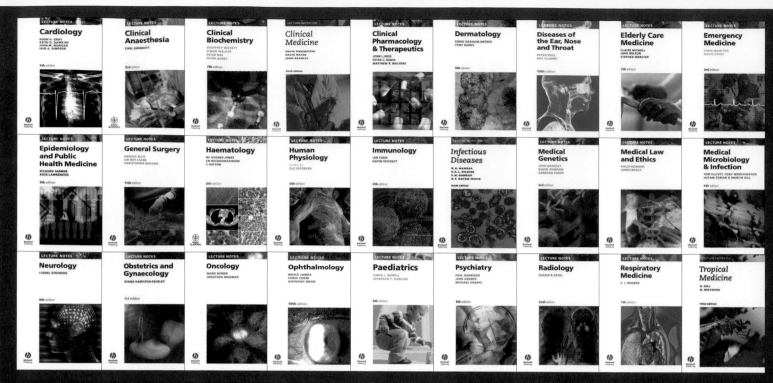
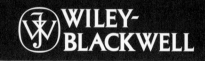

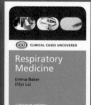
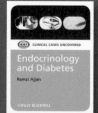
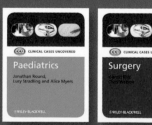
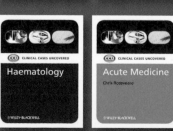
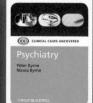
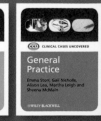
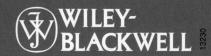